THE

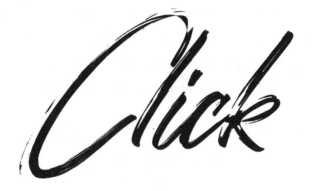

How I Lost 90 Pounds
& Finally Found Fitness...

After 60

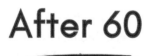

Sharon Odom

This book is for informational purposes only, it is not intended to take the place of advice from trained medical professionals. You should consult a doctor before starting any weight loss program. The author takes no responsibility for any possible consequences arising from the application of any of the advice or information in this book.

Published by:
GeoLocal Media Group, Inc.
Houston, TX

Cover Photography: Isaiah Fling

ISBN: 978-0-9718971-1-3

First Edition

10 9 8 7 6 5 4 3 2 1

Dedicated to my beloved Mother

Beulah L. Odom

&

my children

Kiata, Isaiah, Mariah and Sierra

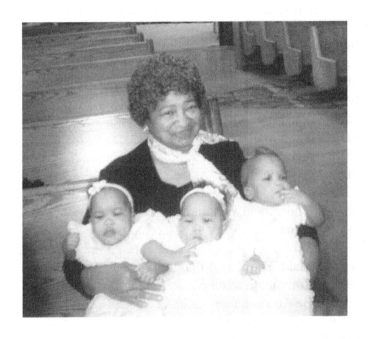

Visit

and download your **FREE** quickstart

guide to **"Living the Click"**

Table of Contents

Introduction

First of all, this is not a diet book. If you're looking for some revolutionary breakthrough technique that will allow you to magically shed pounds without any effort, stop looking. It does not exist in this or any other book.

Here's the biggest complaint about most weight loss books – "There's nothing new here." or "I knew all of this already."

There's a reason for that... because there IS no secret to losing weight. You know all that you need to know. There is nothing fresh and new.

Yet every year more diet books are published, and people buy them. Why? Because we're always looking for the magic bullet, hoping against hope that there's an easier way.

Sorry to disappoint you, but there are no shortcuts.

Weight loss is simple. Burn off more calories than you consume. **Eat less. Move more.**

That's it. That's the truth and there's no getting around it. Believe me I've tried.

If you want to learn about nutrition and various weight loss methods, there's plenty of information available at your fingertips, courtesy of Google. Everything you need to know is out there for free. That is not the goal of this book.

I'm not a doctor, I'm a regular person. Everything I've learned about weight loss has been through research. And **plenty** of trial and error. This is my story, how I was finally able to lose 90 pounds and achieve a healthy normal weight... at age 61.

When I started writing this memoir, my only intent was to share what worked for me. I never set out to be a weight loss guru or a coach.

But if my story can help inspire just one person to change their life for the better, it would have been worth the embarrassment of revealing everything I'm about to share with you. There are thousands of weight loss stories, each one unique and personal. This is mine.

Why tell this story?

- First, to hopefully inspire others on the other side of 40, 50 and beyond – it's not too late. It IS possible! You can lose weight and keep it off, at any age.

- Second, to encourage you to create your own customized eating and exercise plan – a sustainable lifestyle that you can maintain... for life.

- And finally, to hold myself accountable and make sure I don't put the weight back on, that would be too embarrassing.

PART I:

222.5 LBS? REALLY?

N obody wakes up one day weighing 222.5 pounds out of the blue, there's always a story. Here's mine.

Early Days

I'll start at the beginning, back when I was a girl growing up in southeast Texas. I wasn't fat, but always had a big butt. No matter what size or age, my butt was proportionally bigger than the rest of me. Hearing that all my life made me think that I was fat. But I wasn't...yet.

In college I fell into the usual late night snacking and partying habit, but being young and active, my weight wasn't really an issue. My butt was still big, but I'd learned to see it as an "asset".

Even after marrying young, having a baby girl, and getting divorced, I didn't really have a weight problem. After graduating from Prairie View A&M University, my daughter Kiki and I left Texas and moved to upstate New York, where we stayed for a couple of years... freezing our asses off!

Yuppie Life in L.A.

After a couple years in Rochester, we moved to Los Angeles. That's when my weight struggles began. Not because I was fat, but because so many women there are ridiculously skinny. I was single, and of course wanted to measure up in the dating pool. So I was constantly fighting my body in the quest to be thin.

After a few years, I finally realized that engineering was not the career for me and went back to school to get my MBA. After graduating from UCLA I settled into a great career, working with computers.

In my mid-thirties, my weight started to creep up a little. I'd been out of grad school for a couple years, had a full-time job and didn't have as much time for exercise as I'd had as a student. Life in the big city was stressful, and food was my comfort.

I still exercised on a regular basis – lots of roller skating, walks on the beach, and lunchtime strolls with my good friend Andrea.

But as I've learned the hard way, you can easily "out-eat" your exercise. We might walk 3 miles on the beach, then stop at a café for drinks and dinner, or have a couple slices of New York style pizza. I never bothered to figure out the nutritional value of anything. And I always rewarded myself with a large frozen yogurt no matter what.

So yes, I fell into the trap of thinking that because I exercised a lot I could eat as much as I wanted. No. Exercise by itself is not going to cut it, although it does give you some leeway.

In the end, even if you don't track it, **your body tracks every morsel without fail.** When the input is consistently greater than the output, the result is a steady march up the scale. Your body is like a bank. It tracks every penny/pound whether you do it or not. You find out the balance when you step on the scale.

The Hilton Head Metabolism Diet

When my weight hit 175, I was like, "Oh, hell no!". I had to do something. That's when Andrea turned me onto The Hilton Head Metabolism Diet. The concept was to eat small meals throughout the day and to exercise 20 minutes after eating, which gives your metabolism a boost. It came with a defined set of menus and recipes.

I started in the summer of 1987 and followed the plan to the letter. There wasn't much variety or substitution, but I was determined. You can do anything for a short period of time, and I was determined to get down to 130 pounds.

Every morning I would get up early enough to eat breakfast, then go for a walk before going to work. After a quick lunch I'd take a 20 minute walk. And every day after dinner I would go for a long walk in Fox Hills Park.

Every time I ate anything, I'd try to go for a walk. I didn't go out with friends much because it was too hard to follow the diet when away from home. If it wasn't on the plan, I didn't eat it.

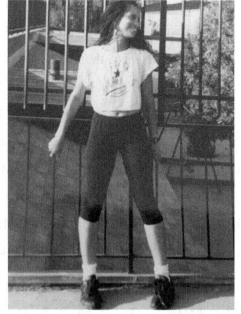

It worked, just like any restrictive diet will if you follow it. Those 45 pounds melted away and I felt wonderful. I couldn't believe that I weighed 130 pounds. I may have even gotten to 129 pounds ...for one day.

Like "queen for a day", **the girl on the fence** was thin for a day...

Well, like any "diet", I couldn't eat that way forever. As soon as I achieved my goal, I went back to eating the foods I loved, and the weight started to creep back up.

Little by little, I gained most of it back.

Years went by, and I was still fighting with my weight. It was a constant struggle to keep it under control. Typical yo-yo dieter.

Marriage & Motherhood...TRIPLETS!

In 1995 I settled down and got married. Before my wedding I worked like crazy to lose weight so I would look good in my dress. On that day I weighed about 150 pounds and felt pretty good.

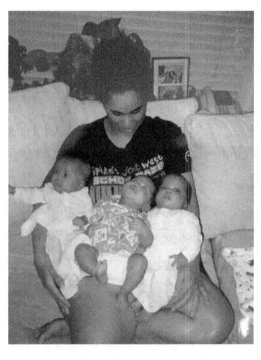

Then, in 1996 I got pregnant ... **with triplets**. For once, having big hips was a good thing – being my size was great for bearing multiple children at once.

I sailed through the pregnancy with very few complications and went on bed rest at 20 weeks, which is normal for higher order multiples.

At the time I was working for The Walt Disney Company in Burbank, and was lucky enough to be able to take 8 months off to have the babies and recover. Thank you Mickey Mouse! A bit of trivia – I once played White Rabbit at Disneyland.

The triplets were born at almost 36 weeks, excellent for 3 babies, and each weighed about 5 pounds.

Before I got too big to see past my stomach, I remember getting on the scale and seeing **233 pounds**.

I weighed a bit more by the time they were born, but that's the number that stuck in my mind as *my highest weight ever.*

I wasn't having any more kids after that, so never did I imagine getting anywhere **NEAR** that number again.

After the babies were born, I never lost all the weight, mostly because of the stress.

Marriage, triplet motherhood and a full-time job left very little time for exercise. Forget that nonsense about running after babies keeping you fit. It does not. After they go to bed, there's plenty of time to stuff your face.

When the kids were 2, we moved to a neighborhood with a Weight Watchers nearby. I kinda liked WW because you could eat anything within reason. Even though they disguise the calorie counting by calling it points or whatever, it really is calories in vs. calories out.

I weighed about 200 pounds when I started, and managed to lose maybe 15-20 pounds, but couldn't seem to get below 180. I didn't like going to meetings or following a particular eating program. The yo-yoing continued.

Back to Texas

When the triplets were 5, we moved to Texas to be near my family. This ushered in a new period of stress. My husband stayed in Los Angeles for the first few months, and my oldest daughter Kiki was out on her own. So I was on triplet duty alone, while starting a new online marketing venture.

Plus, it's hot as hell in Houston most of the year. When it's not hot, it's allergy season. Or raining. So I wasn't getting much exercise. The weight started to creep back up.

A few more years went by and before I knew it, my weight was back in the 200s. All the pictures of me during this period included one or more children in front of me. I was thankful when they got bigger and taller. My weight kept fluctuating, up and down. I would have some short term success every now and then, but couldn't seem to get any traction.

Working from home gave me the flexibility to exercise during the day, so I started going to the community gym several times a week to walk on the treadmill. But I always had to get back to my desk or pick up the kids from school.

The Treadmill Desk

In October 2006 I was watching an episode of Primetime 20/20 and saw an interview with Dr. James Levine. But it wasn't the usual sit down conversation. No, he was walking slowly on a **treadmill** that was positioned **under a standing desk**, while he talked about the concept of Non-Exercise Activity Thermogenesis or NEAT.

This was a light bulb moment for me! I knew as soon as I saw it that a treadmill desk would work for me, especially since I worked at home and liked to walk!

I immediately bought a heavy duty treadmill, and placed the leaf from our dining room table across the rails. It fit perfectly. I put my laptop there and started walking while I worked.

It was *perfect*. Every day I walked 2 or 3 miles without thinking about it, and the weight started melting away. This encouraged me to eat better.

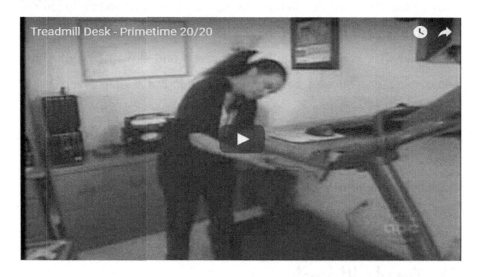

By July 2007 I was under 200 pounds. I started keeping a daily journal about that time and kept track of my weight there.

I continued to lose weight, and was happy to have discovered something that worked so well. I wrote blog posts about the treadmill desk, along with regular updates on my weight loss.

In 2008, Primetime 20/20 found my treadmill desk story online, and came out to interview me for a follow up on their original segment with Dr. Levine. By then my weight was down to 169 pounds.

It was the triplets' 11ᵗʰ birthday on the day that Helaine Tabicoff and a 2 person ABC camera crew came out to the house. We got the kids out of school for a couple hours so they could appear in the segment.

The ABC crew was at the house for **FIVE HOURS**, filming me driving to school to pick up the kids, serving them a snack, walking at the treadmill desk, Helaine interviewing me, etc. They call that "B-roll" footage, and they shot a bunch of it that day.

Guess what? It all ended up on the cutting room floor, condensed to **24 SECONDS**.

The kids were pissed. You could see their pictures in the

background here and there, but other than that, they did not appear in the final televised segment. Here's a picture of us with Helaine and the ABC camera crew.

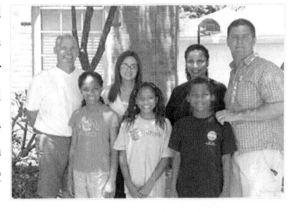

My 24 seconds of fame aired on Primetime 20/20 in August 2008. You can see the video on www.SharonOdom.com or search YouTube for: **Treadmill Desk Primetime 20/20**.

The Body Lift

After having triplets, my midsection had stretched way beyond what any amount of exercise could repair. Even after losing the weight, I had a spare tire permanently hanging around my waist and hated it. No matter how much weight I lost or how much I exercised, it was *never* going to go away.

By the time the Primetime 20/20 spot aired in 2008, I had lost 50 pounds. Thanks to the treadmill desk, I thought my weight struggles were over. To reward myself for having lost the weight, I decided to have a body lift in August 2008.

It sounds so simple, right? Like a tummy tuck or mommy makeover. All of these cute little terms for what really is MAJOR SURGERY! Not trying to scare anybody but this stuff is serious. Potentially life threatening.

Just to be clear, this type of body contouring surgery is **not** a quick way to lose weight. It's usually the ONLY way to get rid of excess skin *after* you've lost a lot of weight. It's not a shortcut to weight loss! No reputable doctor will use surgery to remove a substantial amount of weight from your body. There is **no** substitute for losing weight from the inside out. If so, there would be no overweight rich people.

With a body lift, excess skin is surgically removed from your stomach and hips, anywhere from 5-15 pounds worth. After the surgical team removes the excess skin, you're stitched back together. This is a **360 degree incision**, all around your *entire body.*

If you decide you want a body lift or any other type of body contouring, be SURE to get a board certified plastic surgeon who has extensive experience doing this type of surgery. My doctor was a top expert and well worth **every penny**. This is *not* the time to pinch pennies and go for the cheapest option.

The recovery period is long and painful at first. You have to sleep in a recliner for awhile, and wear compression garments around the clock for months. And you have a lovely scar that goes all around your body.

But I'm **1000% thrilled** with the results, and have *no regrets* about getting the surgery. I would do it again in a heartbeat. Believe me, my stomach would *not* be this flat without the body lift.

Anyway, the results can be fantastic once you get through recovery. But don't be fooled by those simple sounding terms – it's major surgery, it hurts, and it can kill you. I was lucky. There have been many others who didn't live to tell the tale.

My cousin Theresa asked me why on earth would I have such a surgery. I wonder the same thing about people who climb Mount Everest, jump out of planes, or anything else that others might deem a needless risk. To each his own.

Yes, anytime you go under the knife there's a chance something could go wrong. But for me and countless others who decide to have restorative or elective surgery, it's a calculated risk vs. reward.

Besides, my body had always tolerated anesthesia well. And most important, I had done my homework, and had chosen a *world renowned doctor* with hundreds of satisfied, happy, *living* patients.

In October 2008, two months after the body lift, my weight was 158 pounds, the lowest since 1995. I thought that my weight problems were solved forever. You'd think after going through all that, there's no way I'd gain back the weight, right? Wrong.

Life Happens

Being an emotional eater means food is *always* the answer whenever something good OR bad happens in your life. Life was actually pretty good right about this time – I'd sold a website for a nice sum of money and rewarded myself and the family with several wonderful family vacations. We lived in a beautiful house with a pool. We ate out a lot.

Then I started a new website, in a niche I didn't know much about. I spent a lot of money on designers and programmers. My husband lost his job. The stress mounted.

My father passed away, and even though we weren't really close, it stirred up old childhood issues of loss and abandonment. My husband couldn't find a new job. The new website wasn't doing well. The weight started to creep back up.

Mind you, *I was still walking at the treadmill desk every day.* Maybe not as much or for as long, but I never stopped walking. It's just that **my caloric intake exceeded my walking output**. My friend Marina didn't understand it. She's like, you walk all the time, how can you be gaining weight?

Easy. A pound is 3,500 calories. It goes on a lot quicker than it comes off. It takes less than a minute to eat a doughnut but you have to walk over an hour to burn it off. Want a couple slices of pizza? That's another couple hours. Add an ice cream cone. Now you're talking over 4 hours to work it all off. The math is inescapable. There's not enough exercise in the world to overcome the damage your mouth can do in just a few minutes.

I knew the value of food logging and was kinda doing it, but only half assed. But even if *you* don't do it, your body will unfailingly track every calorie that goes into your body.

I became good at avoiding the scale.

In 2011, my weight shot up from 181 to 200. I was mortified. How could this have happened? I was so sure when I weighed 158 that I would NEVER see the 200 mark again, yet here I was.

It would get worse.

Rock Bottom

In 2012 my marriage collapsed. The new website failed. The triplets were 15 years old. We had to sell our house. Their father left the state.

It was the most stressful time of my life, and of course I soothed myself with all manner of food and drink. Lots of it. I still walked at the treadmill desk every day, but no amount of exercise can keep up with out of control eating.

In 2014 my Mother got sick, and was in and out of the hospital a lot. My sister Harrianne handled most of her care thank God, but still it was hard to watch her decline and face the inevitable. I was in denial, sure she would bounce back like always.

When she died on January 15, 2015, I weighed 210. After her funeral I sank into a deep depression, barely functioning. The kids' father returned and helped get them through high school. But when I went off the rails, everyone else did too. It was a very bad time for all of us, and I'm so thankful that we all survived.

As we approached the one year anniversary of Mom's death, I knew something had to change. I was not working much, in a deep funk, and at rock bottom. For everyone's sake, I had to get it together.

On the one year anniversary of Mom's passing, as we stood at her grave, **something clicked**. It felt so real, it was almost palpable … like the flipping of a switch. It was time to reboot my life.

The Long Road Back

I chose February 1st 2016 as my transformation start date. That gave me the last half of January to mentally prepare. I cannot stress this enough – weight loss is **MENTAL**. You must be ready, and have an **inner knowing** that overrides anything that you see in the mirror or on the scale.

On Monday February 1st, I finally faced the scale -- 222.5 pounds. Wait … what??? **The last time I weighed that much, I was pregnant with triplets!** I couldn't believe I'd done this to myself, and felt so embarrassed.

It would have been easy to feel overwhelmed by the enormity of that big ass number, but like all journeys, you have to start with the first step.

I had already beat myself up about it plenty along the way, every time I looked in the mirror. All I felt that day was resolve and gratitude for the opportunity to live life to the fullest. It certainly wasn't happening at 222.5 pounds.

At 5'6" and 222.5 lbs, my **BMI** (Body Mass Index) was 35.9 – **very obese**. Thankfully I hadn't developed any obesity related health problems.

I set an end goal of 148 pounds, exactly 1/3 of my body weight, which would result in a BMI of 23.8. I figured it would take a year, 6.2 pounds per month – totally doable.

What would be different from before? After all, I had lost weight before.

For one thing, I knew better than to follow any plan that deprived me of my favorite foods. **THAT** would not work for me. Here's what I had finally realized:

The way you eat has to be a way of life, <u>not</u> a diet that you start and stop.

Think "diet" the NOUN, *not* the verb.

"Diets" in the traditional sense do not work *long term* because they are temporary. Any weight you lose on a diet will usually find its way back to you.

The word diet has gotten a bad rap and we need to change that. Throw out the word "diet" as something you *do*. Forget about it being something you go on and off.

<u>"Diet" is what you eat and drink</u>. Period.

If you look at diet as a verb, well, you can do anything for a short time and lose weight. So technically, yes, **diets do work.** But most are not sustainable. You must find a way of eating that you can do forever.

How long can you eat boiled eggs or cabbage soup?

Depriving yourself of your favorite foods will make you miserable and unhappy. That's no way to live. For me, life is not worth living if I can't have my favorite foods, whatever they happen to be at the moment.

Also I knew that **food logging was critical for me.** My niece Raye had turned me onto **MyFitnessPal**, so I decided to use it to track every calorie I consumed. It also tracks the nutritional breakdown – carbs, fat, protein, etc. Everyone has to figure out what works best for them. There is no one size fits all, it has to be tailored for each person. Tracking food and exercise was crucial for me.

The other thing that was different – **a conscious decision to monitor and limit carbs.** I'd been resisting this idea for years, not wanting to give up bread and pasta and cake. But everything I read and my own experience had convinced me that I had to reduce the amount of empty carbs I consumed. **Not <u>eliminate</u> – monitor and reduce.**

But that would come later. I didn't start off limiting carbs, just limiting calories and **creating the necessary deficit required to start losing**. More about this later...

I knew that all calories weren't created equal, and that I'd have to tackle the carbs/fat/protein ratios at some point. The good news is, you can still have cake and ice cream and anything else that you love. Just not as much as before.

Fortunately, thanks to my treadmill desk, I already had an exercise program that worked for me. It was a way of life at this point, as natural as breathing.

So yes, exercise was already a habit, it was the nutrition side that I had to get under control. Working out is great, but it's the food choices you make during the rest of the day that will determine weight loss success.

The Importance of Mindset

You cannot begin this journey until you're ready. REALLY ready, not half assed "I'll try and see what happens" ready. No, you have to KNOW. You must have that inner knowing, inner seeing, YOU at your ideal weight. The "nothing but death can keep you from it" type of vision. I finally had that.

And you have to recognize the ***dirty truth about losing weight and keeping it off*** … that when you get "there", you have to keep doing what you did to get there. That had never sunk in before, but ***I finally got it.***

Gratitude

Finally, a central theme in my life was **gratitude**.

Grateful to have had my mother for as long as I did.

Grateful to my sister Harri for taking care of Mom while I dealt with the crap going on in my life.

Grateful to my children for growing up to be good, responsible young adults.

Grateful to God for giving me a second chance. I looked at every day as a chance to start anew.

I didn't have a name for it yet, I just knew that it was time to reinvent myself, create a new vision for my life and for my children. I knew that I could not help them if I didn't first help myself.

I forgave myself for everything I had ever done to hurt myself or those I love, whether it was done consciously or subconsciously.

Again, **losing weight is more mental than physical.** Someone who truly loves themselves will find it easier to lose weight. I had to learn to love myself all over again, because it was obvious that I had lost that somewhere along the way.

From then on, I adopted the practice of extreme introspection and self-love. It was the best thing I could do for myself and my family.

Ready. Set. Go.

I was ready. And determined. With age comes the awareness of how precious time is, and how fleeting. Tomorrow is promised to no one. And if you think about it, we know **for sure** that time is limited and **WILL** run out. The time to do anything is NOW.

I was 60 years old, standing at my mother's grave, and I knew it like I'd never known it before – it was now or never. Something *clicked* for me, and I KNEW that **this was it**.

This time would be different because of the lessons I'd learned along the way.

I knew better than to follow any diet, or to deprive myself of anything I wanted. I was **NOT** giving up any of my favorite foods.

I had a plan. It was not a diet, it was a lifestyle.

Now it was time to ... just do it!

My journey began on February 1, 2016.

PART II:

MY WEIGHT LOSS JOURNEY

Year 1 – The First 74.5 Pounds

This is a month by month account of how I went from 222.5 to 148 pounds over a period of 12 months – a loss of 74.5 pounds. Much of this was taken directly from my journal. It's more detailed in the beginning, then tapers off as it became a way of life and the weight came off slower. During this time I was living with my 19 year old triplets, Isaiah, Mariah & Sierra, and their father, Mark.

Notes:
- My initial goal was to lose about 2 pounds a week, which equals 7,000 calories. Realistically weight doesn't come off in a

straight line, so I figured 6-7 pounds a month would be doable.

- Month end weight is actually from the next day, the 1st of the next month.

- Daily weigh-ins don't work for me, although at first I did get on the scale every day. Sunday was my usual weigh-in day.

- **I wrote this book while walking at my treadmill desk.** I know it's not feasible for everyone to have a treadmill desk, but I truly believe your weight loss journey would be so much easier if you have a way to exercise at home, preferably something you enjoy. Whether it's a stationary bike or rowing machine, whatever you will **use on a regular basis** to move your body will work. If you like to walk and have enough room, you might want to build your own treadmill desk. Maybe you already have a treadmill sitting in the corner. Dust it off, remove the boxes, and find somewhere else to hang those clothes! Actually treadmills have come a long way since 2006. Some will fold up and out of the way or slide under the sofa, so it might not take up as much room as you'd think.

- I worked at home so was able to walk during the day. This isn't possible for many people but shouldn't be an excuse – how many hours a day do you spend watching TV, talking on the phone, or surfing the web? Those can be spent walking at your treadmill desk. Or riding your exercise bike. Whatever works for you.

- Status and Lessons Learned are summarized at the end of most months.

Month 1 – February 2016

I like starting things on the first of the month and/or on Mondays, so when I saw that February 1st fell on a Monday, I knew it was the perfect day to begin my transformation. I actually felt excited and looked forward to the journey. Sort of.

First, a visit to the scale. Naked, first thing in the morning after getting rid of every possible ounce from both inside and out. That included the Fitbit and hair scrunchies.

Weight: 222.5 pounds. Ouch. I knew it was going to be bad, but damn! The last time I was anywhere *near* that number, at least I had 3 babies to show for it a few weeks later …

Next, selfie body shots. Oh this was so painful. For some reason I cut off my head in many pics, which I blamed on

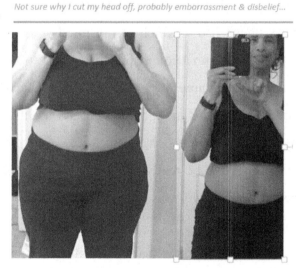

Not sure why I cut my head off, probably embarrassment & disbelief...

February 1, 2016 – 222.5 pounds

the fact that taking selfies was new to me.

C'mon now. I'm no psychologist but have had enough therapy to know there was something else behind that – perhaps a way of disassociating myself from the fat girl in the mirror.

I put those two pics together to prove that yes, that was definitely me in February 2016. Also took my measurements. More horror.

- Bust – 45"

- Waist – 39"

- Hips – 51"

- Thighs – 29"/30"

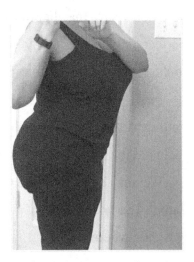

Ok, once I faced the scale and knew the damage, I finalized my plan: **Lose 1/3 my body weight, 74.5 pounds, which would put me at 148 pounds.** That's under 150 – which in my mind was skinny – with a couple pounds wiggle room.

Next, I updated my settings in MyFitnessPal (MFP), which I'd started using back in April 2015, but wasn't mentally ready so didn't keep it up.

You have to be really **really** ready to do this. That's what January was about. No way was I starting on January 1st. I needed the entire month to prepare!

Anyway, MFP said that based on my current and goal weights, my daily calorie intake shouldn't exceed 1550. I linked the Fitbit to MFP, and set it so that the apps would exchange data and sync automatically.

The Plan
Based on all that, here's the "lifestyle" plan I came up with ...

- Track everything I eat or drink in MFP. *Everything*.

- Track all exercise with Fitbit, always synced with MFP.

- **Create a deficit of 1,000 calories per day,** through a combination of eating less and exercising more, with a goal of losing 2 pounds a week.

- Aim to consume about 30% protein, 40% carbs, and 30% fats (at least 80% of the time).

- Nothing was off limits and **I had to love (or at least like) everything I consume.**

- That was it. Nothing else to remember. Complete freedom to have anything I wanted as long as I followed those rules.

The First Few Weeks

I don't believe in weighing myself every day, but for the first couple weeks that's exactly what I did. At the beginning your body sheds water weight, and I *needed* that encouragement.

I lost 5 pounds in the first week, YES! Sure, it was probably water weight but still, it felt good to see the number going down!

Because I worked at home and had been walking at a treadmill desk since 2006, exercise wasn't an issue for me – I just had to keep it up, maybe pick up the pace a bit and walk at a higher incline. So every day I walked at the treadmill while working, checking email, on the phone, or watching TV. Usually 2 to 3 hours or more.

Once I started religiously logging every calorie, it became very clear how all of that weight had found its way onto my body. It wasn't so much WHAT I was eating, it was the AMOUNT. I had been eating way too much. Duh.

Yeah that's obvious, but not until you see it laid out calorie by calorie do you realize how much you're actually eating. That's the value of food logging. You can't fool yourself into thinking you didn't eat that much or just had a few bites. No, you ate the whole thing and it showed up on your body. Food logging tells the truth!

So it wasn't a matter of radically changing my eating habits. It's not like I was a junk food junkie, I was just eating too much. If your body needs 2,000 calories a day to maintain itself and you give it 2.500 every day, that extra 500 calories is stored as fat. Do that every day and you'll gain 1 pound every week. That adds up quickly.

This is a universal truth – calories work the same way in every country, every culture. Eat too many of them and you get fat.

Once I got serious about monitoring and limiting calories, the weight started to melt away... slowly. That's the worst thing about weight loss. It's slow as hell. It comes off a lot slower than it goes on.

Gaining weight is easy, subtle, and way more enjoyable than losing. You can fool yourself for awhile into thinking your clothes have shrunk or whatever. Then one day you're like, "OMG I got fat overnight!" No, you've been getting bigger all along, you just finally woke up and faced the music.

That's what happened to me. I faced the scale, got the message and DECIDED to do something about it – *click*!

Daily Life

Being self employed with sort of grown children meant that I didn't have to go out into the world every day and sit at a desk, which was great. My kids all worked, went to school, and were reasonably self sufficient. So I didn't have to cook dinner for them unless I wanted to. Another plus. So really all I had to do was keep my eye on the prize, stay focused and make sure I got my steps in every day.

For the first month it was a matter of getting my food intake under control and reining in my appetite. Listen, I love to eat, and realized early on that me following a restricted diet was *never* going to happen. That's why traditional diets had never worked for me. Don't tell me what I can and can't eat, that's a recipe for disaster.

So for me, the currency with which I bought all the food I wanted to eat was ... exercise. And that's exactly what I did – walked at the treadmill desk off and on every day.

Day after day, I tracked the calories consumed vs. expended, and made sure that at the end of the day there was a caloric deficit of 1,000 calories, or at least as close as I could get.

That's really the gist of what I did, and if you take nothing else from this book, remember this: **Weight loss boils down to calories in vs. calories out**.

Yes, I know – weighing and measuring food, counting calories, being mindful of portion control – none of that is sexy. Well neither is being overweight. Eat less and move more. Or, my version – **eat well and move a lot**.

Everything in Moderation ... Yeah, Right

I did have my moments of weakness. A few weeks in, my daughter Mariah made a cake and I wanted some. This was the first big test of my "everything in moderation" rule.

Well 1/16th of a cake is not much, but that's all I could afford calorie wise, and you know what? It was just enough to satisfy me. I put a bit of icing on it and it was delicious! That was a revelation – it doesn't take as much as you think to satisfy a craving.

Sometimes I ate more than I should. I read somewhere that you need to change things up, not let your body get used to a set amount of food or exercise. Sounded good to me, the perfect excuse after eating too much.

Overall I learned to be satisfied with less by savoring the food I did eat. I paid attention to how food tasted. I ate off of small plates. Slowly. No more scarfing down anything mindlessly. I truly enjoyed everything I ate.

Weight Loss is a Mind Game

Mentally, I was in a good space. To me it was a mind game. Once the decision was made, there was no way I was going to let anything stand in my way.

But the reality of weight loss sank in – it's painfully slow. My mojo was back, but it would take my body awhile to catch up. I knew that as long as I stayed the course, the weight would eventually go away.

After a few weeks I really got into it. I settled into my new lifestyle, enjoyed everything I ate, and was encouraged by the scale's downward trajectory. It felt like I was finally getting myself together, little by little getting more organized and focused. Using MFP religiously and getting control of my caloric intake gave me a tremendous sense of power.

I also began to feel like the best investment I could make was in myself – fresh braids, nails done, new clothes, whatever it took to make myself feel good again. And as long as I lost at least ONE pound a week, I felt happy, like I could do this indefinitely.

And that's the key. You must be able to enjoy life along the way, so that there's no rush to get "there". Because once you get "there" you have to keep going.

I decided to schedule a getaway trip to L.A. to reward myself for losing 40 pounds. Mind you, I had only lost 6 pounds at this point. But I knew – inner knowing, inner seeing – that by August I'd weigh 185 or less. I felt confident of that in a way I'd never felt before, and looked forward to long walks on the beach.

Be Sure to Eat Enough

After the first 5-6 pounds melted away, things slowed down to a crawl. Yes those first few pounds are encouraging, but don't think that will be an ongoing trend. Eventually all the water weight is gone and you're down to what feels like a snail's pace.

One day in the 3rd week of February, I jumped on the scale and it said 218.0 – WTF??? I had barely eaten 1,200 calories the day before and walked for several hours, so I just *knew* it would show a big weight loss. NO! As a matter of fact it was up a pound. I was pissed.

Here's the lesson: **if your body thinks it's starving, it will hold on to every ounce**. Eat enough or pay the price. Don't get cute and start skipping meals, thinking that will accelerate your weight loss. It won't. Also keep in mind that after a hard workout, your body might retain water for "rebuilding".

Right about this time is when I gave up Lean Cuisines and most frozen pre-packaged meals. These "convenience" meals no longer tasted good. Too many carbs. Too much sodium. Not enough protein or nutrients. I threw them all out.

Near the end of the month I took a quick peek at the scale -- 214.0!!!! Never thought I'd be so excited about such a big ass number, but yes! Something was working, probably a combination of things.

I thought about having lost only one pound a week after the initial 5 pounds and realized that wasn't so bad. I was never really hungry, didn't feel deprived, and could eat whatever I wanted, just not as much as before. This was doable!

February Status

- Starting Weight – 222.5
- Ending Weight – 214.5
- Pounds Lost – 8

Notes & Lessons Learned

- It's important to eat enough. **If your body thinks it's starving,**

it will hold onto every ounce. Skipping too many meals to lose weight faster will backfire.

- Water consumption is important, it definitely helps with weight loss. If you don't like water by itself, disguise it in the form of green tea or flavor your water. Sure it would be better to drink pure water, but this way is better than nothing. Whatever it takes to get that water into your body.

- I realized that spending money on facial products, new clothes and yes, even a trip to LA – these are all important. I needed to nourish and spoil myself in healthy ways, which helped me to stick with my eating program and keep losing weight.

- I tried meditation and found it hard to stay focused, my mind kept wandering. Then I discovered walking meditation and liked it way better than sitting meditation. The rhythm of the walking can put you into a trance almost.

- I researched green tea, and decided to try Matcha green tea. It's the powder form and has more benefits than a tea bag.

- I started thinking of the next step, resistance training. Researched ways of doing weight training without lifting weights. Looked into resistance training for people who hate lifting weights. Hope springs eternal, I was still hoping for some way to build muscle without actually picking up weights...

Month 2 – March 2016

One month into my journey I had lost 8 pounds – not too bad! It doesn't sound like a lot, but do this for 12 months and that's 96 pounds gone. Most overweight people think that weight comes off way too slowly. We're impatient to see the results when we're doing all the right things, but what about when we were eating whatever we wanted?

Weight gain doesn't happen overnight, it takes time to put on a lot of pounds. It just happens to be more enjoyable than losing it. We enjoy the first part, so what makes us think we can get off scot free on the other end? Life doesn't work that way. It's pay now or pay later. Pay then or pay now. Either way, you have to pay the piper at some point.

Whatever. My March 1st starting weight was 214.5, and I did not record it in MFP because my last entry was 214.0 and I would NOT allow the needle the go upwards. Maybe it was a bit irrational on my part but everybody is allowed to be irrational about something. For me, this was it. NEVER record a weight gain in MFP. (Eventually I got over this...life happens, weight goes up and down. It's normal.)

Whoosh Bounce Hold

On March 5th I went out to dinner with my cousin Daryl, who loves to eat and doesn't give a whit about calories. He chose the restaurant, some out of the way place with no salads on the menu. That's real life, you will be in situations like that. I had banked my calories beforehand by eating very little during the day and walking a lot.

Dinner was great! I enjoyed it immensely, but was mindful of everything I ate and took pictures of the food before we ate. I was able to splurge a bit, then get right back on the program. There was no nutritional info available for any of the dishes, but I entered my best guesses in MFP and overestimated everything just to be on the safe side.

The next day I peeked at the scale – 215.0. Not bad, now that I knew about the **whoosh-bounce-hold** cycle: a big loss one week, followed by a small bounce back, a pound or two, followed by holding relatively steady for another week or two.

I had researched weight loss plateaus out of a growing sense of frustration – the weight was coming off very slooooowly, little by little. I wanted a flood, not a trickle!

Well, weight loss comes in fits and starts. For one thing, your weight can fluctuate several pounds every day, whether you're trying to lose weight or not. A big meal, lots of carbs, salty snacks, water intake, constipation, heavy exercise – any of these can cause your weight to go up temporarily. A pound is 3,500 calories, so as long as you didn't eat 17.500 calories in one day, you didn't really gain 5 pounds overnight.

Also, even if you're eating and exercising in a way that creates a caloric deficit, the scale may not budge. That's because fat doesn't burn up and disappear the way we imagine it does.

No, you exhale most of it as carbon dioxide. In the meantime, fat cells shrink, at which point water often swoops in to take its place. And you know how heavy water is! So, the fat is gone, water has taken its place, but the scale doesn't know the difference between fat and water. This is why the scale is not always the most accurate indicator of fitness.

Anyway, these water filled fat pockets can persist for **days** or even *weeks*. The scale may not reflect a weight loss, or even worse, it may show a weight **GAIN**. This can be very demoralizing and cause you to say, "What the hell, I may as well eat." Don't do it! Train yourself not to panic. Trust the process and be patient. Stick to your plan like glue.

The Whoosh Effect

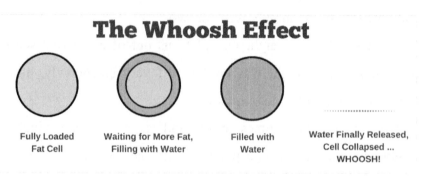

| Fully Loaded Fat Cell | Waiting for More Fat, Filling with Water | Filled with Water | Water Finally Released, Cell Collapsed ... WHOOSH! |

Eventually, the water stores will suddenly release, almost overnight and – **WHOOSH!** No, you didn't really lose 4 pounds in one day. It's an accumulation of your previous days or weeks worth of losses finally being reflected on the scale. *Booyah!* Then, the cycle starts all over again.

For more information on the whoosh effect, search the internet or the MyFitnessPal community forums, you'll find plenty of evidence that it *is* a thing.

10 Pounds Gone!

On March 13th I weighed 212.5 pounds – that's 10 pounds gone, for an average of 1.67 pounds per week.

Not too shabby, especially since I didn't feel deprived. Well, I still hadn't had pizza yet, but felt confident I could handle it now.

A few notes from that time:

- I started to not like meat that much, not even chicken really, mostly fish.

- For the first time, I felt a bit skinnier! Maybe it takes 10 pounds to feel a difference.

- One day when I tried to complete the MFP entry, the app fussed at me for not eating enough, refused to post it to my news feed or give a 5 week weight loss projection. Too funny!

Eating Hacks

Here are some tricks I discovered this month:

- I ordered a **stovetop smoker** to reward myself for being so good. It quickly became my favorite kitchen appliance, great for making smoked tilapia and shrimp. Tilapia thaws in just a few minutes, has so much protein, and tastes so good! It's definitely become my "go to" meal for a quick infusion of protein that satisfies. We ate it with steamed spinach or 50/50 salad/spinach mix with a sprinkling of shredded cheese and light ranch dressing. Yum!

- Realized I need to stop eating so much yogurt – too much dairy plus it has way too many carbs.

- Carbs really do count. Much as I hated the idea, I knew I had to find a way to reduce carbs. I used to put an entire banana in the smoothie, then reduced it to a couple small slices, if at all. Not total deprivation, just being aware and mindful, and make sure it's worth it. Started to slowly get rid of the high carb favorites and find others. It was tough though because most of my favorite foods were high in carbs. Arrgh!

- Came up with the perfect iced tea recipe – 1 teabag of green pomegranate decaf tea and 6 bags of decaf green tea – brew all 7 bags together in electric tea kettle, sweeten with stevia and chill. Very tasty way to get your water down!

Finally toward the end of the month, a WHOOSH! Weight 208.0 – YES! Moving in the right direction! Only 9 pounds from my next goal – the 190s. It was working! I had lost 14.5 pounds in 2 months and definitely felt thinner!

March Status
- Starting Weight – 214.5
- Ending Weight – 208.0
- Pounds Lost – 6.5
- Total Lost – 14.5 in 2 months

Notes & Lessons Learned
- Learned how to deal with weight lost plateaus – it's called the "Whoosh-bounce-hold" effect
- I read somewhere that sleep is important for weight loss. Uh oh. I struggle with insomnia a LOT and often feel tired and

lethargic from lack of sleep. Could this be hindering my weight loss? Figured out how to wear Fitbit at night - very loosely on my arm. *(Only did this for a couple months to see my sleep patterns. Not good.)*

- So happy I'd finally figured out a way to eat that kept me happy AND still able to lose weight! It really felt different this time, like all I had to do was stay the course and it would lead me to 148 pounds.

- The stovetop smoker is MAGIC!

- Stevia became my go to sweetener, no more splenda or any other fake sweetener or sugar.

- Researched how to exercise while intermittent fasting.

Month 3 – April 2016

Two months into the journey, my weight was down 14.5 pounds – 208.0. So far so good. I had managed enough projects for Disney to know the value of breaking a large project into manageable bite sized chunks, otherwise the enormity of it can be overwhelming. That's definitely the case when you set out to lose almost 75 pounds. The goal seems so far away.

So I set up some intermediate goals, with rewards small and large along the way to keep myself motivated:

- Next weight goal - 200.0, then 199.5.

- Then...185-186 -- new BMI threshold (from obese to overweight) – L.A. here I come!

- Also at that point I will be HALFWAY to my weight goal of 148 pounds...
- Then, 170, which is what I weighed 8 years ago...
- Then, 158, my lowest weight since the triplets were born.
- THEN every pound after that until I hit 150, and finally...
- 148.5!!!!!

Love My Fitbit

I'd read that 10,000 steps a day is what we should aim for, and immediately set out to do that, using Fitbit to keep track. But there was a problem. I'd walk for HOURS and still wouldn't get there.

So I joined the Fitbit forums and searched for an answer. It turns out that others had experienced the same thing. Fitbit is designed to be worn on the wrist, and I learned that it doesn't count treadmill steps correctly because the tracking is based on movement. Well, I was staying in the same spot all day. So THAT'S why it was taking so long to get to 10,000 steps!

Then I found a suggestion in the community forums – try it on your ankle. The next day I put the Fitbit around my ankle and BOOYAH! It was like magic – all my steps got counted and I was up to 10,000 in less than 2 hours! Soon I was routinely hitting almost 20,000 steps. I was *very* happy to have found that discussion.

Something else I learned from the forums – walking outside is way more strenuous than treadmill steps. After studying the Fitbit stats, it became clear that was true – the intensity of the exercise is definitely higher outdoors than on a treadmill. This encouraged me to walk outdoors more often.

Once I started posting in the forums and became a member of the community, people started inviting me to participate in Fitbit challenges. Daily Showdowns, Workweek Hustles, Weekend Warriors, Adventure Races, Marathons … there are always challenges going on that you can participate in if you wish.

Before I knew it, my Fitbit was humming with activity. I already had a strong walk habit, this just made it a bit more fun. My Fitbit "clique" developed quite naturally and is still going strong today.

There's also a community tab where people share their accomplishments, awards and pictures across various groups (Hiking, strength training, weight loss, etc.). If you get a Fitbit, be sure to add me as your friend and let's do some challenges together. My Fitbit ID is: **kalona3**

There are other fitness trackers out there, but because my daughter gave me a Fitbit, that's the one I use. MFP syncs with other fitness trackers, and of course there are other food logging programs out there as well.

But MFP and Fitbit are the ones that I use and love them both! Both of the apps are free, the only cost is the Fitbit tracker itself. In case it's not abundantly clear, the combination of MFP and Fitbit has been a huge part of my success.

"Nothing Off Limits" Put to the Test

About mid-April my weight was down to 206.0 – 16.5 pounds lost in 10 weeks. Staying on that pace would put me right at 185 or less by the end of July. I booked the trip to L.A., which meant I had 3 months to lose 20 pounds. That was a nice big juicy carrot pulling me forward...

But after being strict about eating well for over 2 months, I was feeling a bit deprived of my favorite foods. Now it was time to put the "nothing off limits" policy to the test.

One day I made chicken enchiladas, one of the triplets' favorite meals. I ate 2 of them, with rice and beans, light sour cream and pico de gallo. Yummy!!!! It was my main meal of the day and totally worth all the walking I had to do to "earn" it.

A few days later, my cousin Theresa brought over one of MY favorite meals – fried drum from our favorite hole-in-the-wall fish market. The meal comes with french fries and bread, but I ate only the fish, nothing else. Guess what? I enjoyed it immensely, and was so happy to finally have fried drum that I didn't even miss the fries.

During this time I grew sick of smoothies and came up with a new breakfast – 1/2 English muffin, fried egg, 2 slices bacon and ½ slice Tillamook cheese. It was delicious! This became a permanent part of my breakfast rotation, except eventually it became 1 slice of bacon and no cheese.

Overall, I began to relax a bit and allow myself more food choices. Remember, this had to be a **way of life**, and that meant fried fish, enchiladas and anything else I wanted, within reason.

The biggest difference this time was *awareness*. By entering everything into MFP, I knew exactly how many calories were going in. And after having whatever it was, I went right back to eating tilapia and spinach. This was the 80-20 rule in effect, as it is in almost every other area of our lives.

I also started to be more conscious about the connection between feelings, food, and hunger. Was I really hungry or just bored? I learned to eat less, but truly savor and enjoy every bite more.

Mindful Eating & Mindless Exercise

It was about this time that I really started to look at this as a game of "me vs. me". Here are the questions I wrestled with:

- How much **enjoyment** and **nourishment** could I get out of the calories I consumed vs. how much exercise I had to do to earn them?

- Where in my daily "diet" could I shave off some calories and carbs without missing them or feeling deprived?

- How could I increase the number of calories burned without increasing the time spent exercising?

I decided to increase my treadmill walking speed to get my heart rate up into cardio zone. Walking at 1.1 mph barely got my heart rate up, so I needed to up the pace.

But it's a tricky thing – you can't walk too fast, otherwise you can't really do any computer work. I learned to increase the pace to 1.5 mph or more while watching TV or talking on the phone, etc. If I needed to type, the pace was 1.3 mph or slower, depending on how much typing I needed to do.

Another thing – I tried a new mix of fruit in my smoothies once I saw that strawberries have less carbs than blueberries or raspberries.

Once I started reading labels closely, I saw how many carbs I had been consuming in every area, especially smoothies.

I learned to pre-measure the fruit into sandwich bags so that they were ready to use on smoothie days, and I knew exactly how much was going into the smoothie. There's no substitute for a good kitchen scale!

One day I realized I'd forgotten to put banana slices in the smoothie and didn't really miss it. That was a quick way to shave off 8-10 carbs.

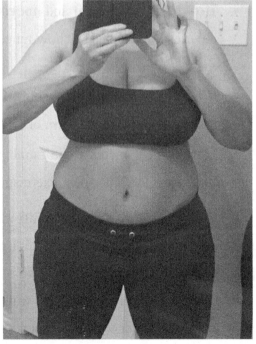

18 Pounds in 3 Months

On April 24th my weight was 205.0 – 17.5 pounds in 12 weeks. Time for a new status picture! You could definitely see the difference.

By the end of April I weighed 204.5 —YES!!! Ok, it was only a 3.5 pound weight loss, but still, **18 pounds in 3 months.**

I didn't feel deprived and felt my health getting better every day. Besides, I just KNEW that a whoosh was coming soon...

April Status:

- Starting Weight – 208.0

- Ending Weight – 204.5

- Pounds Lost – 3.5 lbs

- Total Lost – 18 pounds in 3 months

Notes & Lessons Learned

- According to the BMI calculator, my next major milestone was 185 lbs – still overweight but no longer obese. From there it was 30 pounds to **normal weight**. In my mind I was already there, my body just had to catch up.

- Bought an electric tea kettle to brew large amounts of green tea. Tried several different teapots, finally settled on one.

- Started cooking fresh vegetables instead of frozen. Fresh tastes *way* better.

- Tried a couple different protein bars. They were ok but none tasted that great. Decided to stick with real food and only use them for emergency nourishment.

- Tried Matcha green tea, started including it in my smoothies.

Month 4 – May 2016

I started May at 204.5, so down 18 pounds after 3 months -- YAY!

I felt pretty good about my progress. It felt like a nice, steady, DOABLE pace. And I never felt hungry, unlike previous "dieting" experiences.

Within a couple days I got the long awaited "whoosh" and weighed 203.0 on May 3rd. The whoosh phase is wonderful! I was only 1/2 pound away from having lost 20 pounds.

By Mother's Day the scale said 201.0. The 190s were in sight! As ridiculous as it may sound, this is how you monkey bar from one goal to the next. Keep going! Every goal is only a few pounds away. Reward yourself at every turn.

Food Boredom *Is* a Thing

We all tend to eat the same things over and over. That goes double when trying to lose weight. You know the drill ... grilled chicken breast and broccoli. Or in my case, tilapia and spinach. That stuff gets boring AF very quickly. Variety is the spice of life. You need different meals to keep things interesting.

I definitely got tired of smoothies, and experimented with other breakfast foods. I tried egg whites, but found that I prefer the whole egg, yolk and all.

We used the stovetop smoker a LOT, at least twice a week. My family got tired of it, but everybody was old enough to fix what they wanted so they always had that option. Oddly enough, as much as they complained, the kids would eat everything I cooked. Everybody was eating healthier.

Fitbit Foolishness

The Fitbit challenges definitely made me start walking more, but for a minute I got caught up in the competition, doing stupid stuff like jiggling my foot while resting to rack up more steps or using a lower incline on the TM so I could walk longer. I realized what I was doing and stopped that foolishness immediately. The goal was to lose weight, not win challenges!

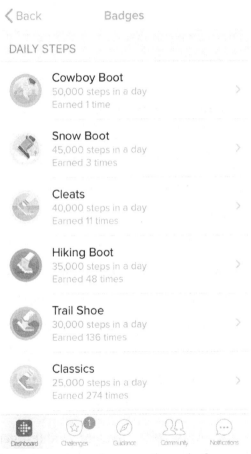

One of my Fitbit friends said he got caught up and started eating too much because of the challenges. I was very careful not to eat much more than before, so the additional exercise went toward losing weight.

But overall, as long as I kept my eye on the ball, the Fitbit challenges were a lot of fun, and definitely pushed me further than I ever would have gone by myself.

One day my Fitbit friends invited me to a 40K challenge – 40,000 steps in one day. As I got close to the end, they pushed me to do just 5,000 more steps. Then another 5K.

That was my one and only 50,000 step day, something I don't ever plan to do again. But I did get 3 new Fitbit badges that day – 40K, 45K and 50K.

Waiting for the Whoosh

Remember how the cycle starts over after each whoosh? After a quick 3-4 pound weight drop at the beginning of the month, my body decided to replenish the water stores again. The scale did not budge, for weeks.

I was sooooo close to 199.5 that I could taste it! I started walking a lot more, which only caused my body to hold onto even more water.

One day I jumped on the scale and it said 202.5, up 1.5 pounds. Not true of course, I just accepted it as the "bounce" part of "whoosh-bounce-hold" and kept right on stepping.

Here's a series of food diary entries that show the torturous nature of waiting for the whoosh....

- **May 20th** – Weight: 200.0 – getting closer! Definitely feeling my 22.5 pound weight loss now, hey! Triplets turned 19 today and we went out to eat; it's no big deal to eat out now, amazing...

- **May 22nd** – Weight: 200.0 … still, but it's about to go WHOOSH any day now!!!

- **May 23rd** – still 200.0 but the whoosh is coming! Totally lost track of time, was shocked to find out I'd walked 200 minutes. The TM is magic…

- **May 24th** – weight still 200.0, the whoosh is coming. Tried spiralizer to make noodles out of zucchini, turned out great. Zucchini pasta allows you to get the spaghetti feel without all the carbs in pasta.

- **May 25th** – still 200.0 dammit! No more visits to the scale til Sunday. Took it easy today, didn't walk as much, my body needed some rest. Discovered that when I walk a lot, like 30k steps or more, my body seems to retain water, maybe to help build muscle. I read somewhere that a hard workout causes the body to retain water for rebuilding.

- **May 27th** – 199.0 FINALLY! I wasn't going to weigh myself again til Sunday but couldn't help it — hopped on the scale, 199.0!!! Finally out of the 200s, in the 190s – YAY!!!

- **May 31st** – weight 197.5 – YES, the whoosh is in effect!

May Status
- Starting Weight – 204.5
- Ending Weight – 197.5
- Pounds Lost – 7 lbs
- Total Lost – 25 pounds in 4 months

Notes & Lessons Learned

- Don't go food shopping on an empty stomach…ever.

- Really got into the Fitbit challenges this month. These friendly competitions really pushed me to a new level of exercise. Having a group of people to regularly step with is just another motivation tool. Although I walked plenty before, the camaraderie and competition definitely spurred me to greater heights.

- Started wearing size XL shirts, no more 2XLs!

- Watched "The Secret" DVD, always good to have a refresher. *See it. Believe it. Achieve it.*

- Tried a spiralizer to make noodles out of zucchini, the zucchini pasta turned out great! It allows you to get the spaghetti feel without all the carbs in pasta. Wasn't sure how to cook it, sauteed it a bit, found out later from my daughter that steaming it in microwave is the way to go. Need to buy 2, one zucchini is not enough.

Month 5 – June 2016

On Wednesday June 1st my weight was 197.5. I had just set that goal and almost overnight, BAM! 25 pounds in 4 months. That's about 1.5 pounds per week.

Sure, it would be nice if the weight would come off a wee bit faster, but I had to remind myself that this wasn't a race. Slow and steady weight loss has a much better chance of being permanent. The key is to not feel deprived and be able to eat anything you want, within reason.

Based on current weight loss and projections, I calculated it would take about a year to reach goal.

Can't Beat the Heat

Living in southeast Texas growing up and in Houston since 2003, you'd think I'd be used to the ungodly summer heat by now. No. Every year it seems to get hotter and hotter. I can't believe I used to run around and play in this hot mess as a child. After living 20+ years in Los Angeles, long gone was the acclimation of my childhood years, replaced by fond memories of year round hiking and walks on the beaches of Southern California.

So yeah, summers suck in Houston. All I wanted to do was stay inside my nice air conditioned house. As a result, my outdoor walks all but stopped. Unless I woke up early and went out first thing, it wasn't going to happen. It doesn't cool off until late evening, so most of my walking was done inside on the treadmill.

I also craved stuff like Greek yogurt, frozen yogurt, yogurt bars, watermelon. Cheese and crackers. Wine and fruit. Carbs, carbs and more carbs. My weight loss slowed down as a result.

Funny thing though in the winter I don't have any issues. But then again, winters are very mild in Texas. I'll bet some people in colder climates have similar issues during winter months. Something to be mindful of – seasonal weight loss challenges.

Mid-June Update

In mid-June it was time for a new status photo, this time using MFP's Progress Gallery feature. This allows you to show 2 pictures side by side.

Once you hit the 25 pound weight loss mark, something happens. It's enough weight loss for clothes to fit differently. For people to notice. To feel better.

According to the National Heart, Lung and Blood Institute, "losing just

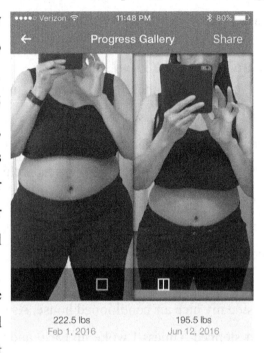

5 to 10 percent of your current weight over 6 months will lower your risk for heart disease and other conditions." Just losing a small of weight can result in lower levels of cholesterol and fatty triglycerides and decreased blood pressure.

So yeah, having lost well over 10% of my weight, I felt very happy with my progress at this point. I loved being able to eat all of my favorites – maybe not as much as I wanted, but that was the deal. That's what I had to give up to get to a normal weight.

I'd found an exercise regimen that worked, although I knew that at some point I would have to start strength training to tone up. But for now, the focus was to continue the count downward to 148.

By the end of the month I was down 6 more pounds, in spite of the heat and extra summer carbs!

June Status
- Starting Weight – 197.5
- Ending Weight – 191.5
- Pounds Lost – 6
- Total Lost – 31 lbs in 5 months

Notes & Lessons Learned
- I got better at avoiding carbs, although it's very tough to do in the summer. Looking in the mirror, seeing the pounds melt away, seeing myself looking better, all of that REALLY helped to keep the motivation high.
- I learned to do walking meditation on the TM, way easier than sitting meditation.
- *Really* ready for some better fitting clothes; long t-shirts over leggings is not a good look.

Month 6 – July 2016

After 5 months, my weight was 191.5 – 31 pounds down, 43.5 to go. Only 2 pounds to my next goal, the 180s!

This is what you must do – have short term goals and reward yourself for reaching them. At least that's what worked for me. Every goal was an excuse for a manicure/pedicure, massage, facial, etc. Treat yourself, you deserve it. Later on the rewards got bigger...like a new car!

On July 8th my weight was 189.5. My next goal was 185.0, which would move me from obese to overweight. My plan was to reach that goal by August 5th, when I was leaving for Los Angeles.

Who knew that simply *being overweigh*t would be such an exciting **important** distinction?

Family Reunion Time

On July 15th the kids and I traveled from Houston to Baton Rouge, Louisiana for a 2 day family reunion. At this point my weight was still 189.5 (another whoosh-bounce-hold cycle). I was a bit apprehensive about being around all that good food. Would I be able to resist? Down home southern cooking is laden with lard, sugar, and carbs for days – hardly what you'd call healthy eating.

Well it wasn't as hard as I thought. For one thing, there's plenty of barbecue – that's nothing but protein! Nobody says you have to eat the potato salad, yams, cornbread, cakes and pies. I filled my plate with chicken and focused on talking to family members I hadn't seen in 2 years. Nobody really noticed or cared.

That's when it dawned on me. It's just food. The important thing about a reunion is connecting with family members, not eating! I wasn't even tempted that much. Doing the mental calculation was enough for me to pass up almost everything: 1 big slice of cake = 2 hours of walking – NO THANKS! I did have a bit of peach cobbler though, and enjoyed every bite.

Every day when we got back to the hotel, I would jump onto the treadmill in the gym to finish up my 10K steps for the day. For some reason I thought I'd feel deprived of all that good home cooking. Nope. I wasn't into the food at all, but immensely enjoyed what I did eat, and it was a wonderful reunion.

Back to Houston from Baton Rouge

We got back to Houston on Sunday night. On Monday morning I jumped onto the scale, anxious to see what the damage would be, and was shocked to see 188.0!

WHAT? That means I had lost weight in spite of going to a family reunion! I think that's when I really really got it – yes, I could live like this for the rest of my life...

Check out the status pic, you can really see the difference between 222.5 and 188.0. Notice that more

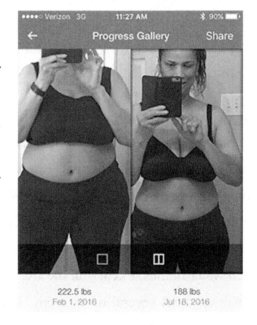

of my face is visible and there's even a hint of a smile...

No Longer Obese!

The week after the reunion, I lost 3 more pounds, bringing my weight to 185.0. At 5'6", my BMI was 29.9 – **NO LONGER OBESE!!!** Still overweight, yes, but obese, **no**!

After losing 37.5 pounds, I was over halfway to my 74.5 pound weight loss goal. Excitement doesn't begin to describe my feelings at this point. I was *in the zone* now, and was not going to stop until the scale said 154.5 or less - NORMAL weight, no longer overweight. I hadn't felt this certain since ... well, never.

I was aiming for 148, but remembered that my butt started looking a little flat at 158, after the body lift. I couldn't remember the last time I'd weighed less than 150, and began to wonder how I'd look at that size. I knew I'd have to do weight training at some point, but wasn't mentally ready yet.

Plantar Fasciitis – Ouch!

I started having pain in the heel and arches of both feet, which turned out to be plantar fasciitis. From reading about it on the Fitbit forums, it was pretty common, and also really painful. I decided to limit my steps to 20K steps a day until it got better.

The best remedy is icing, which I did several times a day using frozen water bottles. I kept 4 in the freezer at all times, and would roll my feet on them several times a day. It seems we use ice to reduce inflammation in all areas of the body -- head, ankle, knees, and feet.

My cousin Rose suggested some plantar faciitis exercises, which helped some, but icing is really the only thing that brought relief. I tried to take it easy on the treadmill by decreasing the incline, but it cut my calorie expenditure in half. I guess walking uphill really *does* burn the calories.

Then I found some plantar fasciitis socks on Amazon, sort of compression garments for your feet. I put them on top of my regular socks and they hugged the feet tightly. I don't know why this worked, but the pain definitely decreased. Between the icing and the amazing socks, within a few weeks the pain was barely noticeable.

And by the end of the month, I had lost another 2.5 pounds, bringing me to 182.5 for a total of 40 pounds lost in 6 months. Getting there!

July Status

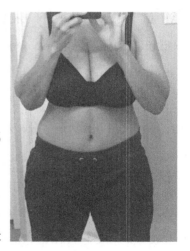

- Starting Weight – 191.5
- Ending Weight – 182.5
- Pounds Lost – 9
- Total Lost – 40 lbs in 6 months

Notes & Lessons Learned

- I stopped wearing the Fitbit at night, much better to sleep free.
- Started tracking outdoor walks with Fitbit; the app generates cool looking reports.
- If you ever get plantar faciitis, get some compression socks,

they work!

Month 7 – August 2016

August 1st marked 6 months since my weight loss journey began and I was ecstatic to record 182.5 in MFP – that's 40 pounds in 6 months!

I took new status pictures and also updated my measurements:

- Bust – 38 (-7 inches)

- Waist: 34 (-5 inches)

- Hips – 45 (-7 inches)

All in all, I felt pretty pleased with my progress, and published several blog posts about my weight loss on www.SharonOdom.com.

One of the biggest "ah ha" moments – **I finally learned how to eat out.** Here's the thing: ***There's no reason to get something extravagant or fattening just because it's a special occasion.*** You're *not* wasting the occasion by eating something healthy!

That was a **big** "click" for me. I learned to enjoy the experience of eating out by **focusing on friends and family,** not the food. Just in time too, with the L.A. trip coming up!

Off to Los Angeles!

On August 5th, I left for Los Angeles weighing 181.0, which was 4 pounds under my goal of 185. Sweet!

I spent the next 3 weeks visiting all of my favorite places and hanging out with my old friends from grad school and my early yuppie days. Every day there was a walk or hike somewhere like ...

Kenny Hahn Park – My friend Linnette and I walked from our buddy Ray's house to Kenny Hahn park. It was about a mile away, down and up hills. Then a few more miles up and down hills in the park before heading back. I knew the last mile was going to be all uphill and I was dead tired. I almost let Linnette go get the car, but knew I'd feel like a punk so gutted it out and dragged my ass up that hill. I've never been so tired in my life! When we got back I laid down for a long nap. That walk was definitely beyond my level of endurance, and it wiped me out for the rest of the day.

Runyon Canyon – this has always been one of my favorite hiking spots, right down the street from the Hollywood Bowl with a perfect view of the Hollywood sign. We parked at the top and hiked a couple miles to the bottom, then started back up. I encouraged Linnette to go the steeper route – she was about 40 pounds lighter than me and I didn't want to hold her back. No, honestly I didn't want to have to walk faster to keep up with her. She went up the expert path and had a great workout – the steep steps even scared her a little. She was so happy! In the meantime, I trudged up the regular path at my own pace, carrying my extra 40 pounds in peace. I was very happy to get back to the top, whew! Afterwards we went to Quickie's, which brought back fond memories from when my family in Sherman Oaks. Me and the kids used to go there all the time for pizza and yogurt. Linnette and I ordered a large pizza and ate 2 slices each, it was SO good.

Venice Beach – spent the day walking the strand alone, all the way from Marina Del Rey to the end of Venice Beach and back, about 6 miles. Enjoyed the sights and sounds of the boardwalk, and didn't even want any frozen yogurt.

Manhattan Beach / Ladera Heights – walked the strand from Manhattan Beach to Hermosa Beach and back with my dear friend Andrea. This was about 6 miles, part of it up and down hills to get to and from her house. A few days later we walked all around Ladera Heights, lots of up and down hills, about 5 miles worth.

Del Cerro Park in Palos Verdes – this is a beautiful trail, another one where you start at the top and walk down, down, down. I walked about 2 miles down, then hauled my 180 pounds all the way back to the top. Fitbit registered it as *100 flights of steps.* I was SO tired by the time I got back that I could barely drive home! Outdoor steps are WAY more strenuous than treadmill steps, that's for sure.

Redondo Pier to Hermosa Pier – parked near the Redondo Beach Pier, walked along the strand all the way to Hermosa Beach Pier and back. That's about 6 miles round trip. No hills this time though...

Eating Out in L.A.

I went out several times with friends for dinner and drinks, and it was easy to eat healthy in health conscious California. I had lots of grilled and blackened salmon, tilapia and chicken. And focused on the experience of being with my friends, not the food. I practiced mindful eating the whole time, but rewarded myself for all the hiking and beach walking too.

Back to Texas

I returned to Houston at the end of August, feeling somewhat apprehensive about all those dinners and drinks. And my step count was way down on most days. Imagine my surprise to discover I had lost 3.5 pounds and was in the 170s!!!

August Status

- Starting Weight – 182.5
- Ending Weight – 177.5
- Pounds Lost – 5
- Total Lost – 45 pounds in 6 months

Notes & Lessons Learned

- Even without my handy TM I still managed to lose a few pounds on vacation! I didn't walk as many steps as usual, but the steps I did were *strenuous* – outdoors, and mostly up and down some serious hills. This is definitely a case of quality vs. quantity – 10,000 steps in L.A. is way more work than 20,000 steps indoors on the treadmill.

- Being **ready for a change** is the essence of *The Click* – when you're ready, you can make anything happen. Who knew that I could spend 3 weeks in L.A., enjoy myself thoroughly every day, and lose weight while doing it?

- I practiced mindful eating, and ate whatever I wanted within reason. I made sure to take pictures of meals before eating them since a lot of it was stuff I didn't usually have. This way I could add it to MFP later.

- I didn't weigh myself for 3 weeks because each scale is different, and you should weigh yourself on the same scale every time for consistency. When I got home and weighed myself, I was shocked to discover I had lost weight, especially after everything I ate.

- It felt good to get rid of all those big ass t-shirts – tossed them all out and kept purging.

Month 8 – September 2016

Ok, 7 months in and I was down to 177.5 – that's 45 pounds gone.

A 5 pound weight loss in September would put me at 172.5, just in time for my birthday. So that became my next goal...

Here's the thing about losing weight. You think it's going to solve all your problems. That once you're thin, your life will be perfect.

That's not true, and this was the month I recognized it.

Early in September, it hit me. My kids were grown and would soon be moving out on their own. My ex-husband and I had a good relationship, but we were no longer married. Eventually we would all go our separate ways, and then what?

Yes I was on my way to being thin, but I was also 60 years old. No amount of weight loss can turn back the clock, and we live in a youth obsessed society. What would I do with myself once I reached goal?

These were the dark thoughts of September. In the past that would have been enough to send me diving into the nearest vanilla pudding cake.

Not this time. I'd come too far to sabotage myself now. I had to stay the course. In the meantime, I had 5 pounds to lose by my 61st birthday. Instead of stuffing my face, I went for a walk. And when I got back I watched "The Secret" – it's always good to get a refresher on "The Law of Attraction".

50 Pounds Gone!

My goal for September was to lose 5 pounds and get to 172.5. I couldn't change my age or what my kids did, but THAT I could control.

On September 4th I weighed 175.0 - WHAT? Checked it several times, it was 175.0 each time. I wasn't dehydrated or starving so took it as my real weight, and recorded it in MFP. That was 47.5 pounds gone, well within my weight loss goal of 50 pounds by October 1st.

I really loved the way I ate, and didn't feel deprived at all. I wasn't eating carbs that often, but really enjoyed them when I did indulge.

Instagram Is GREAT for Weight Loss

At this point I started posting to Instagram (**@sharoneodom**) and SO wish that I'd been doing it all along. IG is PERFECT for weight loss transformations. People are so encouraging and accepting. If you're just getting started, I urge you, **post to Instagram!** Start on Day 1, it's great for accountability.

By now I definitely felt skinnier, and found myself interacting with random people more, smiling and exchanging comments.

It's amazing – the smaller I got, the more visible I became. It made me realize how much overweight people are ignored in our society. Sad but true. All of a sudden people were talking to me more, noticing me more. The only thing that had changed was my weight. Or was it? Maybe I was more outgoing because I felt better about myself.

The Road to 172.5

At this point my sole focus was on losing 5 pounds to reach 172.5 by my birthday. I got really stingy with the calories, and totally focused on that 50 pound weight loss goal.

One day I made enchiladas and ate only ONE – and it was just as satisfying as having 2. I skipped the rice and beans, and didn't even miss them.

I learned to eat off of tiny plates, which makes a little food look like a LOT.

By mid-September, I was at 174.0. So close!

From that point on, I checked my weight almost daily. I normally wouldn't do that, but I had to make sure I was on track to reach 172.5!

On September 26th I weighed 173.0 – only a HALF pound to go! My birthday goal was right there!

Finally, on September 29th it happened – 172.5! That's 50 pounds in 8 months. **FIFTY POUNDS!!!**

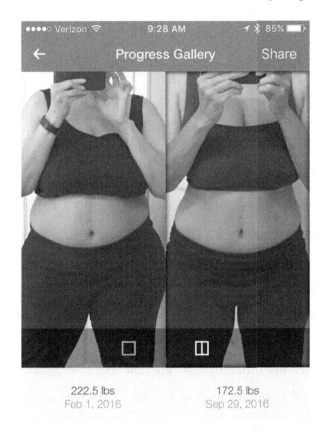

| 222.5 lbs | 172.5 lbs |
| Feb 1, 2016 | Sep 29, 2016 |

September Status

- Starting Weight – 177.5

- Ending Weight: – 172.5

- Pounds Lost – 5 lbs

- Total Lost – 50 pounds in 8 months

Notes & Lessons Learned

- So happy to have figured out how to lose weight in a way that's healthy, yet doesn't deprive me of anything. I enjoy what I eat and have found a way of exercising that works for me. The combination of MFP and Fitbit works and I'm very grateful to have found it.

- Eat off of small plates – it makes a little look like a LOT!

- I found some black capris that were too tight when I went to LA. Now they felt very comfortable. It's so much fun to go shopping in your own closet...

Month 9 – October 2016

On October 1st I weighed 172.5, exactly 50 pounds less than when I had started this journey 8 months earlier.

I celebrated my birthday knowing that no matter what, I would stay the course and continue to lose weight. This was a commitment, a promise to myself that I would not break. To celebrate, we had New York style pizza from my favorite place and it was delicious!

Time for Some New Threads

After purging my closet of the big mumu looking shirts, plus all the 2X and XL tops and bottoms, the clothes racks were looking a bit sparse. I was down to almost nothing that fit. It was time for some new threads – not too many, just enough to get me through to 148 pounds. And to reward myself for all that hard work!

I went shopping and bought some size 14 jeans that fit perfectly. What a great feeling to finally be *done* with the plus sizes! I also got a few sports bras, tank tops and exercise pants. Everything was cheap or on sale since I didn't plan to wear them for too long...

I also got rid of lots of old Dallas Cowboys shirts, all way too big and some were faded to boot. I asked myself, "Why the hell am I hanging onto this crap?"

Some people say you should keep at least one momento from your fat days as a reminder. Not me. Nope. All gone.

Vision for Remainder of 2016

Every now and then you need to stop and reassess. This often happens in your birthday month. My goal and vision for the remainder of the year was to keep up the slow and steady weight loss so that by January 2017, I'd be within striking distance of my 148 pound goal. In my mind's eye, I could already *see* that number on the scale: 148.0 in big red numbers on the black background. And it was only 24.5 pounds away...

As a sidenote … it's funny, I appreciate my body so much more NOW than when I was younger! Seems like we are so critical of ourselves sometimes. Now I look in the mirror and think, hmmm, not so bad.

People Starting To Notice

One day my daughter Sierra said, "Mommy, have you lost weight?" Ahh, that sweet moment when the people around you start to notice that there's less of you now!

Another day Mariah asked was I eating enough. She thought I had lost too much too fast. Ha!

My kids were used to my weight fluctuations over the years, and I'd been walking at the treadmill desk since 2006. So it probably wasn't obvious at first what was happening. I certainly didn't announce my goal to lose 75 pounds to them or anybody else. Maybe it's because I'd tried and failed so many times before to achieve and maintain a normal weight.

But it certainly did feel good to have my family notice. Even my son Isaiah said something about it, amazing for a teen-aged boy. I also started getting comments here and there from people at the neighborhood park where we walked sometimes.

I tried to downplay it all. I'd lost weight before, and even though I felt like this time was different, that little voice of doubt kept whispering, "What if you can't keep it off?" So as far as I was concerned, the less said about it, the better.

October Whoosh

By mid-October my weight was down to 170.5. I was always surprised when I got on the scale and my weight was down. Not feeling deprived or hungry, I figured it would mean a weight gain.

A few days later, I reached another milestone – 169.5 – WOO HOO! Back in the 160s!!! I was really surprised because I had taken it easy for a few days before. The body really does hold onto water to help rebuild muscles, and I had participated in some long Fitbit challenges recently.

Then just like that, I lost 2 more pounds and weighed 167.5. Ahhh, the thrill of the whoosh. For the rest of the month I was content to bask in the glow of being in the 160s again.

Except, on Halloween for some reason I couldn't focus on anything and felt totally discombobulated... all day. I was totally unfocused and out of sorts, and had to keep reminding myself of "The Secret" ... all day. But that didn't keep me from walking 35K steps – no matter what, at least I accomplished THAT.

October Status

- Starting Weight – 172.5
- Ending Weight – 167.5
- Pounds Lost – 5
- Total Lost – 55 pounds in 9 months

Notes & Lessons Learned

- Having a bad day? No matter what happens, try to get your exercise in, it will make you feel better about not getting anything else done that day.

- In the past when I lost weight, for some reason I would hold on to the old clothes, just in case. After thinking about it, I decided that's really stupid -- *just in case* <u>*what*</u>? That's begging for the weight to come back! Burn those bridges behind you - throw out the fat clothes!

- Budget for a new wardrobe

- I started putting pineapple in smoothies, which gave it a nice flavor.

Month 10 – November 2016

Heading into the holiday months I was on a roll. My weight was 167.5 with a BMI of 27.0. Losing another 13 pounds would put me at a normal weight with a BMI of 24.9!

Like a rock gathering speed going downhill, I decided that *nothing* was going to stop me from reaching my goal. February 1ˢᵗ was only 3 short months away and I could not, **would not** allow the holidays to derail me.

I continued to do Fitbit challenges, including one particularly grueling Workweek Hustle where everybody did at least 35K steps a day for 5 days.

Foodwise, I was sick of smoothies and all other breakfast foods. I tried Ezekiel flat bread for making bacon and egg breakfast burritos. It was ok, but I liked English muffins better.

I also tried steel cut oats, which look like seeds and have to be cooked the old fashioned way, on the stove top. Sweetened with stevia and a bit of honey, they turned out okay, kinda thick and chewy though. Meh.

Believe it or not, I still loved the taste of tilapia in spite of eating it all the time. It helped to have a variety of ways to cook it – smoked, baked, sauteed or grilled. Delicious every time. I tried catfish but it didn't taste good unless it was fried, so that was that. No more catfish for awhile. If I was going to have fried fish, it *had* to be drum!

60 Pounds Gone

One evening in mid-November I realized that I hadn't eaten enough that day. It was not intentional, I simply was preoccupied with a project and forgot to eat. This happens to skinny people all the time but I NEVER expected to utter those words in my life!

Anyway, it was after 9 p.m. when I remembered, way too late to eat anything. The next morning the scale said 162.0 but of course I didn't believe it. Still I was very happy to have arrived at that number – from 222.5 to 162.0 = 60.5 pounds lost. If I could do that, I could do *anything*. By now I really believed it, that nothing was going to stop me from reaching my goal.

A few days went by and I was still at 162.0, which was less than 5 pounds from my all time low weight in recent recorded history. That was 158 after the body lift in 2008.

At this rate I figured I'd be in the 150s by December and very close to 148 pounds by February 1st. As long as my weight was in the vicinity of 148 I wasn't going to sweat the actual date too much. But you know that deep down I *really* wanted to get to 148 pounds by February 1st. The question was, could I lose 8-9 pounds during the thick of the holiday season?

Thanksgiving

On November 22nd the scale said 159.5 but it didn't seem real so I didn't record it. I thought it would jump back up the minute I believed it. You know, the "bounce" part of the whoosh-bounce-hold cycle.

Our Thanksgiving tradition has always been to make seafood

gumbo instead of turkey dinner with all the fixings. We've been doing this ever since the triplets were babies and they love it.

The gumbo tradition definitely worked in my favor – I didn't have to cook mac and cheese, rice, yams and all that other crap. We have plenty of family and friends who make more than enough of all that stuff, and my kids know where to get it if they want it.

As a result, Thanksgiving dinner was no problem at all – I got my steps in early, then we had our usual fun making the gumbo as a family. The good thing about making gumbo now – the kids are actually a big help, unlike when they were little.

Another good thing – gumbo is full of protein, and even though it's usually served over rice, I simply reduced the amount I put in my bowl. It tasted fine with less, and actually turned out to be pretty good with NO rice!

After Thanksgiving, my weight was 160.0, which I considered to be a victory, given my perpetual sweet tooth. Yes, I enjoyed several pieces of cake and pie that found its way back to our kitchen.

To be *that* close to my all time low weight of 158.0, 3 days after Thanksgiving? I was thrilled!

Something Magic

Heading into December, I felt SO good, like I could do ***anything***. Something magic was happening and I just **knew** that my goal was within reach – 148 pounds by Feb 1st.

A 5-6 pound loss in December and 5-6 pounds in January is all it would take. That's 12 pounds over about 9 weeks – totally doable, even though my body needed fewer calories now. I was *so* in the zone as far as exercising and eating right, it wasn't even a question … just do it.

My energy felt a bit low during the last couple days of November so I didn't walk as much, and worked at my "sit down" desk quite a bit. Always listen to your body – if it's tired, it will let you know. Listen. Even if it means not doing all of your steps...

On the last day of November, my weight was still stuck at 160.0. Even though I felt good mentally, I really wasn't eating enough and that's why my body was holding onto the weight. Who ever would have thought that not eating enough would a problem? It was almost laughable.

Anyway, a plateau at 160 pounds is a great problem to have when you weighed 222.5 only 10 months before! The December 1st weigh-in would tell the story.

In the meantime, I felt nothing but HAPPY and GRATEFUL to have been able to lose the weight in a relatively straight line from February through November. I knew my Mom would be happy and proud, and wished she were here to see it.

Gratitude is a BIG part of this. Be grateful for every pound lost, for every breath taken, for every day... in a blink of an eye, it could all be gone. Say "thank you" every day...

November Status

- Starting Weight – 167.5
- Ending Weight – 159.5
- Pounds Lost – 8
- Total Lost – 63 pounds in 10 months

Notes & Lessons Learned

- Be grateful
- End of month measurements:
  - Bust – 38
  - Waist – 33
  - Hips – 42
  - Thighs – 22-23

Month 11 – December 2016

I woke up on December 1st and leapt onto the scale – **159.5!** After weeks at 160.0, this felt real. I recorded it in MFP and took a new picture. That's 63 pounds in 10 months, an average of 6.3 pounds per month.

Ok, it's not the best picture and I don't know where my mind was on this day but hey – **159.5.**

After a breakfast with no dairy, I settled down with tea and ACV. It felt like a cold was coming on, and I had learned to heed the warning signs and not push it. So I took it easy and walked very little.

In the movie Godfather II, Hyman Roth says, **"Health is the most important thing. Not money, not success, not power."**

SO true! **Health is your greatest wealth** … of that I'm sure.

In the 150s For Real

On December 5th my weight was 158.0. WHAT??? Took a picture of it, then did it again to be sure – still 158.0. YES! This was my lowest weight since 2008! Words cannot express the gratitude I felt. It took a few days before I believed it enough to post it to MFP. That's 64.5 lbs gone.

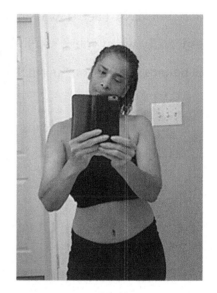

I still wasn't feeling great, so didn't push myself during the next few days. The good thing was, my appetite was off, so I didn't eat much either.

One day I was looking for something to wear to church, and realized I'd reduced myself right out of my entire wardrobe.

Then I tried on some clothes I'd been hanging onto from my 30s and 40s and guess what? They almost all fit, even the sexy red dress from my 1995 honeymoon! And the black lace suit from my Yuppie days in L.A.! I was only about 10 more pounds from where I wanted to be. Unbelievable.

On December 8th I got on the scale and BOOYAH! My weight was 157.5 for the FIRST TIME EVER in recorded history. The lowest was 158 back in 2008, and I couldn't remember when it was less than that, maybe my wedding day in 1995?

Two days later, I was at 156.5. There's nothing like a whoosh, especially when you're so close to goal! That's 66 pounds GONE, only 2 pounds away from normal weight, and less than 10 pounds from goal. YES!

I went shopping for jeans and had to buy a size 12 – amazing!

By then my weight was 155.5 and BMI 25.1 – still overweight by ONE pound.

154.5 – No Longer Overweight!

On December 23rd I got on the scale – 154.5! BMI = 24.9! OMG – no longer overweight! Oh happy day! NORMAL WEIGHT!! Happiness is too small a word to describe how I felt.

Now all I had to do was maintain it through the rest of the holidays and into the new year. That's 68 pounds lost in 11 months, an average of 6.2 lbs per month. I only had to lose 6.5 pounds in January to meet my big goal of losing 74.5 pounds in 12 months – 1/3 my body weight.

By the last day of the year, I'd lost one more pound and ended the year at 153.5 - 69 pounds down. My 148 goal was definitely within sight! Yes, I was in the zone!

December Status

- Starting Weight – 159.5

- Ending Weight: – 153.5

- Pounds Lost – 6

- Total Lost – 69 pounds in 11 months

Notes & Lessons Learned

- Health is the most important thing. Not money, not success, not power. Health is your greatest wealth.

- Ate some skinny girl popcorn, but found that I didn't care for those kind of carbs anymore, it's not worth the uptick in weight every time I eat them.

Month 12 – January 2017

On January 1st my weight was 153.5. At 5'6" that's a BMI of 24.8 – **normal**! I had lost 69 pounds in 11 months, but the goal was 148 by February 1st, so I couldn't rest on my laurels. Fortunately 148 was only 5-1/2 pounds away!

I took my measurements and took a bunch of new status pics.

A few days later, I posted this to Facebook and Instagram...

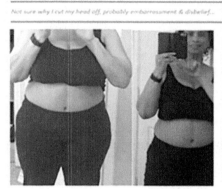
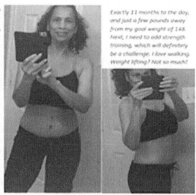

Not sure why I cut my head off, probably embarrassment & disbelief...

Exactly 11 months to the day, and just a few pounds away from my goal weight of 148. Next, I need to add strength training, which will definitely be a challenge. I love walking. Weight lifting? Not so much!

February 1, 2016 – 222.5 pounds   January 1, 2017 – 153.5 pounds

It doesn't matter where you start, anything is possible ... at any age!

www.SharonOdom.com

I'm normally pretty private, and not much of a sharer on social media, so don't ask me why I did it. It's very scary to put yourself out there to be judged – you know how people can be.

Even though the "before" pictures were hella embarrassing, I did it anyway in the hopes of inspiring others, and was happily surprised by the comments of support.

I left it up for a few days, then chickened out and hid it from my Facebook timeline, but left it on Instagram. IG is a very supportive environment for weight loss and fitness transformations, so it felt more comfortable to have it there than on Facebook.

A few days later, another milestone, 152.5 – 70 pounds lost. The countdown to 148 was on!

Another round of purging left my closet practically empty. What a great problem to have! I read somewhere that while you're losing weight you should shop at thrift stores until you reach goal. Then once you've lost all the weight, treat yourself to a new wardrobe.

Time for Strength Training

Once my goal was in sight, it was time to start thinking about strength training. I probably should have started sooner, but honestly I was *not* looking forward to this part.

Walking was easy, something I'd been doing for years. Weight lifting was something else. I'd tried it a few times here and there, thanks to Andrea, but it never quite caught on as a habit. But all of my research told me it was the next step if I wanted to truly get fit.

I was very lucky that gaining all that weight after having the body lift didn't undo the results of that expensive ass surgery. That truly would have been tragic. Now that the weight was gone, it was time to tighten and tone.

There's only one way to do that – resistance training. Good ole weight lifting. Unfortunately there's no shortcut. It can't be bought, otherwise there would be a lot more buff people walking around.

I'm not a gym person, never have been. In order for this to work, there needed to be as few barriers as possible between me and the weights. That meant doing it at home, at least to start.

Being an Amazon Prime member, I had access to a bunch of videos as part of my membership. After reviewing what seemed like hundreds of them, I found some that looked almost doable.

I dug out and dusted off a set of 3-5-8 pound weights that we'd bought years before. I decided to start the next phase of my transformation in February. Like the previous year, I needed the month of January to mentally prepare.

The 140s at Last!

On January 12th the scale said ... **149.0**! WHAT? I was under 150 pounds for the first time in forever! Only **ONE** pound from goal. I could not believe it. To say I felt good would be an understatement. How about skinny, confident and happy? Yep.

On January 15th we observed the 2 year anniversary of Mom's passing. As we stood at her grave, I thought back to that day exactly one year before, how embarrassed and ashamed I felt. I knew Mom would be happy that I'd lost the weight – no more cracks about me sitting on her bed! But I also knew she'd say, "Great! Keep going."

Reached GOAL – 148.0!

On January 20th it happened, the day I had looked forward to for so long -- **I reached my goal weight of 148.0!** And 11 days early at that. It's hard to put my feelings into words. Shock. Awe. Sheer joy. Gratitude.

I took new pictures and measurements – 36-30-40.5, thighs both 22. For some reason I forgot to take a picture in sports bra and bottoms like all the previous status pictures. Duh! Euphoria induced brain fart I guess. Whatever. I was there!

So ...now that I'd made it, what was different from all the other times?

This time I knew better than to relax as if it was over. ***It's never over.*** You have to stay on top of it. Last time I got to 158, I stopped weighing myself, as if I'd arrived and was there to stay. This time I knew better.

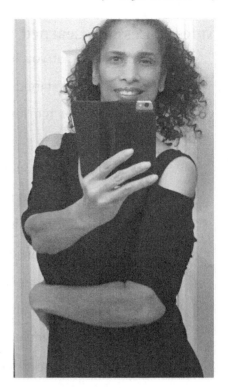

I felt pretty damn good, and wanted to bask in the glow for a bit. But not for too long, the job wasn't done. Next, Phase II – resistance training, which was going to be a huge challenge. For one thing, I hated weight lifting.

Walking was such an ingrained habit that it required no thought or effort. That's not the case with strength training. How was I gonna make myself do this?

I wasn't at all sure about that part, but decided to *intend it*. Put it out to the Universe and see how it would manifest.

January Status

- Starting Weight – 153.5

- Ending Weight – 148.0

- Pounds Lost – 5.5

- **Total Lost – 74.5 pounds in 12 months**

Notes & Lessons Learned

- Did you know that you have bones in your ass? Neither did I. All of a sudden it started to hurt when I sat down or laid in the same position for too long. Apparently this is what happens when your padding is gone. Who knew? Research tailbone pain after weight loss and you'll find many similar stories. It's one of those weird physical changes that can happen when you lose a lot of weight. After awhile the pain goes away...

- I read in a MFP blog article that calories burned measured by a fitness tracker is more accurate than the treadmill readout, so decided to let Fitbit figure it out – one less entry to make. So what if it underestimates calories burned? It makes up for underestimating calories entered into your food tracker. Using the Fitbit calorie estimate saves time – no more manual entries.

- Weight loss slows drastically the closer you get to goal because your body doesn't need as many calories. Gone are the days of big losses and all that excitement.

Year 2 – The Last 15.5 Pounds

Wow, I really did it – lost 74.5 pounds and reached my goal of 148 pounds.

Listen... I've lost weight before, several times. And **each time** it felt like I'd arrived, was done, and could relax.

Now I knew better. Losing weight is only half the battle. The real battle is <u>keeping it off</u>.

This is the hardest lesson to learn.

Whatever it takes to lose weight is what it takes to keep it off.

Sure, you can eat a bit more, but the question is *how much more!* Let's see how *that* went in Year 2.

Sidenote: I continued food logging with MFP and walking

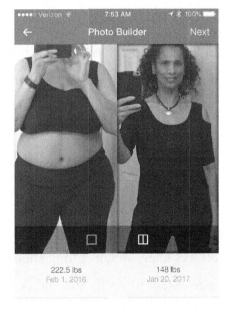

10,000+ steps daily, either on TM or walks outdoors, so no need to talk about that anymore. And I still used Fitbit to track steps and continued to participate in challenges to keep it interesting.

February 2017

The first thing I did after reaching goal was to relax a bit and bask in the glow. Can't a girl have a little fun? I ate more carbs and sweets than usual and just like that, **gained 2 pounds and was back up to 150.** Dammit. I was still walking every day, but had relaxed just a little bit.

That's when I decided to set a new goal of 145 so that a couple pounds wouldn't put me back in the 150s, a place I never wanted to revisit.

I enjoyed my little break, but there was no way in hell I was going to let it creep up any more. That's the key – you have to nip it in the bud – *do not let it get out of hand.*

I immediately went back to smoked tilapia and spinach and cut back on the carbs. It was nice while it lasted, but there is no "there" and you're done ... you have to keep going.

Strength Training

I finally sucked it up and started strength training in February. I always knew weight lifting should be a part of my fitness regimen but didn't want to do it. Still didn't, but it was time to put on my big girl panties and make it happen...

I decided to lift weights 3 times a week. After some trial and error, I settled on a 30 minute strength training video that I could actually finish by The Gymbox, with Ashli. I started out using 3 and 5 pound weights.

After a few sessions with Ashli I decided to check my weight and was shocked: 147.5!

What??? I had lost 2-1/2 pounds just from lifting weights a few times? I decided to keep on training.

From then on, I forced myself to do the strength training workout on Mondays, Wednesdays and Fridays pretty much without fail.

Every now and then I'd try a different workout video for a few minutes but always went back to Ashli. I learned how to mute her voice, turn on subtitles, and play my own music. That made it more interesting at least.

I decided to really commit to weight training, especially after the encouragement my body gave me by losing a few pounds after only a few sessions! That really got my attention because it's the only thing that changed in February.

I had pretty much resigned myself to weighing around 150 pounds. Frankly I was ready to enjoy the fruits of my labor and live a little. So to have my weight drop from 149.5 to 147.5 in a week was amazing, and well worth 90 minutes.

Once I figured out how to play my own music while following Ashli's cues, the time went by pretty fast. I always petered out during the last 5 minutes with the floor work, but kept moving no matter what.

Toward the end of the month I dumped the 3 pound weights and began to use the 5 and 8 pound weights only. OMG my arms really hurt after that! I still wimped out at the end, but learned to keep going.

The combination movements made the 30 minutes go by pretty fast.

Teacake Time

On February 26th Mariah and I went to cousin Harold's to learn how to make teacakes. I would come to regret this day. What was I thinking? Why would I want to learn to make a dessert with butter, sugar, eggs and flour as the main ingredients, while in the middle of my transformation?

Because they taste **so** good, that's why. This was my grandmother's recipe passed down through the years, and if I'm going to eat a dessert, it might as well come from my own kitchen. At least I would know exactly what was in it. Anyway, for better or worse, teacakes became my favorite dessert from that day forward...

February Status

- Starting Weight – 148.0
- Ending Weight – 147.5
- Pounds Lost – 0.5
- Total Lost – 75 lbs since Feb 1, 2016

Notes and Lessons Learned

- Remember, the goal at this point was to only lose a few more pounds to get to 145.0. My primary goal for Year 2 was to tone and strengthen, but because of the surprising results, I continued the monthly status reports through 2017...
- Trying to maintain and not gain or lose is very tricky...

March 2017

By March I'd settled into a routine of strength training 3 times a week. In the morning I would eat fruit and walk on the treadmill for a bit while checking email. Then when I couldn't put it off anymore, I would lift weights for 30 minutes. Then a smoothie and vitamins.

I won't lie – strength training wasn't the most enjoyable part of my day. Most of the time it took every ounce of willpower I had to make myself do it. But gradually it became habit, like showering and brushing my teeth.

I kept bitching about being bored with Ashli, but didn't want to take the time to learn a new routine. This one I could do with the sound muted, playing my own music. A new instructor would require me to pay attention.

I wanted mindless exercise, like the treadmill desk. Ashli was the closest I could come to mindless strength training. I knew that the human body needed to be challenged to get stronger. But I reasoned that a maintenance dose of weight lifting was better than nothing. Besides, I had moved up to 5 and 8 pounds – no more 3 pound weights. Wasn't that enough?

Eventually I decided to try a Jenny Ford workout. She had several videos on Amazon Prime, and even though she was a bit "energizer bunny" like, I could somewhat keep up with her. I would hit the wall at certain parts, especially the lunges, but usually did the whole 37 minutes.

Holding Steady

My weight was holding steady at 147.5, which was amazing considering how many teacakes I ate. We're talking a serious sugar addiction here. I ate them all the time, tracked properly in MFP of course, and had to walk like hell to "pay" for them. I really came to rue the day Harold taught us how to make what he called "Shankleville Crack" – and now I knew why!

By mid-March I'd been lifting weights 3 times a week for a solid month and must admit, it definitely got easier. I still wasn't using the 8 pound weights consistently, so there was lots of room for improvement.

Most of the time I didn't want to do it, and it was a constant struggle to pick up those weights. But I really enjoyed telling everybody that I was lifting weights 3 times a week. That's how I held myself accountable.

Also I noticed muscles developing where there had been only flab before. So I kept going.

Over time a funny thing happened. I began to kinda look forward to it. Other times I would give myself permission to do only the first exercise and quit if I wasn't feeling it. Most of the time I kept going. The 30 minutes would fly by, and a big icy protein smoothie was my reward.

By the 3rd week of March, strength training had become a full fledged habit. I guess it's true what they say – it takes 21 days to create or break a habit. I was still doing the Ashli workout most of the time, with Jenny thrown in every now and then.

One day toward the end of the month I got on the scale and was shocked to see 145.0 - WHAT? I did not believe it. How could that be? I was still eating way too many teacakes, and eating right only half the time, yet here I was only 15 pounds away from my all time low of 130!

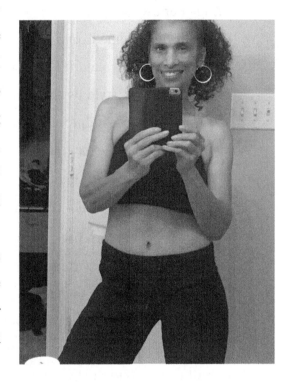

I took new status pics to commemorate. By the end of the month another 1-1/2 pounds had melted away. Unbelievable...

March Status

- Starting Weight – 147.5
- Ending Weight – 143.5
- Pounds Lost – 4
- Total Lost – 79 lbs since Feb 1, 2016

Notes and Lessons Learned

- Not sure why but I **lost 4 pounds this month,** even while eating all those damn teacakes. It ***must*** be the strength training, that had been the only change.

- Bring your own food! I went to a friend's house to hang out and they pulled out some frozen pizza. I was like, oh hell no! If I'm going to spend my calories on pizza, it's going to be the *real* deal – New York style by the slice, fresh out of the oven, not some frozen crap with preservatives. That stuff is nasty! Good thing I had brought some teacakes with me.

- I entered teacake recipe into MFP, which yielded 56 teacakes – 90 calories, 11 carbs and 4 fat grams per 31 gram serving.

- I SO wish I could turn back the hands of time to 1987 when I lost all that weight! I was right there, all I had to do was work to maintain it like I'm doing now. It's so clear to me now that the key to maintenance is ***vigilance***. Why didn't I do this 30 years ago??? Whatever your age, please heed my word. Don't wait til you're 60 to finally get it.

- In retrospect, I really should have started weight training earlier, it would have made the weight come off a bit faster!

April 2017

On April 1ˢᵗ I got up and jumped on the scale: 143.5. **WHAT?** I did NOT believe that number, not when it had been 145.0 only a few days before, and *that* was a sudden drop from 147.5. I was out of teacakes so maybe... nah, something was wrong. Maybe the scale's battery needed changing.

There's no way to sugarcoat it. April was a month of upheaval – the triplets found a 3 bedroom apartment, got approved on their own, and we decided to move. OMG, my babies were leaving home! My ex-husband and I were finally going our separate ways. Being an emotional eater, I ate more than usual, even while keeping up with walking and strength training.

Never lose sight of the fact that your mouth can EASILY out-eat your body's ability to exercise it away.

I definitely ate more in April – anxiety over the impending move, feelings of loss. Stress plays a BIG part in weight loss or the lack thereof...

My weight fluctuated all over the place, from 143.5 down to 141.0 back up to 146. All in one month. At the end of the month it was 143.5, back where I started. I considered that to be a victory! Even when I put in a new battery, the scale still said the same thing so I guess it was accurate. Was it the weight training? It seems like the 140s just flew by.

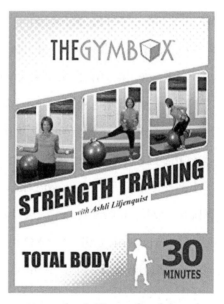

The lesson? Stay the course no matter what! Keep food logging, keep exercising. Keep weight training, even when you don't feel like it. Maintain the vision. Work to keep stress from derailing your weight loss plan...

Weight Lifting is Magic

Wonder of wonders, I began to really enjoy weight lifting. It seemed to go by quicker every time.

By April 5th my weight had dropped to 142.0 -- wow, only 3 pounds from the 130s?! Unreal. Just from strength training? I could not believe it. Weight lifting must be magic. I kept researching other strength training workouts on Amazon Video, but stuck with Ashli and Jenny.

Sometimes I felt tired or low energy and had to force myself to lift weights. Maybe I wouldn't do it full out, or skip the floor work. *But I did something.* No matter what.

You've heard that 90% of life is just showing up. I think that's the case with weight lifting. Just show up and do something.

On April 12th the scale said 141.0 – 2 pounds away from the 130s. Only 12 pounds away from 129! It dawned on me that I could actually get to the 120s if I wanted to. Just... wow!

I tried on size 8 jeans and they were too big. I had to buy a size 6! Unbelievable. I finally had the body I always wanted, at age 61 no less. The irony of it all! It **HAD** to be the weight training.

Toward the end of the month, strength training had become a habit, but I was really bored with Ashli. This would become a running joke...

Because of all the teacakes, I'd gained back the pounds I lost earlier in the month. Once the teacakes were gone, it was time to get back to 141, or even better go for 139! Could I do it? Did I WANT to do it? How bad did I want it?

April Status

- Starting Weight – 143.5
- Ending Weight – 143.5
- Pounds Lost – 0
- Total Lost – 79 lbs since Feb 1, 2016

Notes & Lessons Learned

- This is maintenance. It's not glamorous. The thrill and excitement of big weight drops is gone. You're not even looking for that when you approach the scale. No, you want to make sure you haven't **gained** weight. If so, you have to nip it in the bud. Get your ass back in gear the next day! **This is for life, it's not a diet you start and stop!**

- I was quite surprised to find myself in the low 140s. The irony is that my original goal was 148, then 145, but because of weight training, here I was only a few pounds away from the 130s!

- I started eating pistachios as snacks, sometimes even for breakfast. Experimented with different foods to see how my body would react to added calories, and gained a couple pounds as a result. This is all part of the balance of maintenance, something I had NEVER experienced before.

Why? Because with previous "diets", as soon as I hit goal, I went back to eating like before and gained the weight back, that's why!

- I still loved smoked/sauteed tilapia and spinach, but looked for other things to eat so I wouldn't get bored. Another tasty favorite is California Pizza Kitchen Chopped Salad – visit www.SharonOdom.com or search Google for the recipe, it's delicious!

May 2017

This was a really tough month, in every possible way. Moving sucks under the best of circumstances, and this one was even worse. It signaled the end of our lives together as a family unit. The triplets turned 20 on May 20th and 11 days later we moved.

Emotionally I was all over the place. Not to mention the actual work and stress of moving. We were dividing our household into 3 parts – theirs, mine and his. It's a wonder I didn't crumble, but I had come too far to fall off the wagon now.

Besides, all of my fat clothes were gone. I had no choice but to stay the course. My goal for the month was simple – make it through without gaining weight. Maintain, not gain.

My weight was 143.5, which was a happy surprise considering all of the stress induced snacking. After coming this far, even if I gained a few pounds, I thought I'd be able to climb back onto the wagon. This month would be the true test of all that resolve.

Are Thin People Treated Better?

One day I went to the grocery store wearing a "What's Cardio" t-shirt. It was an ordinary day, but for some reason I got lots of greetings and offers from the staff to help find stuff. Was I more approachable now, did I smile more? Or are "thin" people treated better? It's probably a combination of both. I definitely remember feeling somewhat invisible when I weighed over 200 pounds.

Another day I went for a walk at the neighborhood park and saw one of the regulars walking his dog. He gave me a high five, said I look good and asked how much had I lost. When I told him 80 pounds he was like, whoa.

Think of the enormity of that number. You know when you check a suitcase at the airport how hard it is to heave that sucker onto the scale? Now think about carrying that much weight – if not more – around with you *every minute of every day.* It's amazing when you think about it. Yet we do this every day without thinking about it.

Moving Chaos

I continued with my daily walks and strength training, even amid the growing chaos of moving. At times like this, you rely on habit to get you through. I even managed to do a Jenny Ford workout several times, all the way through, only missing a few push-ups and lunges.

I also started to post to Instagram more, and really wished I'd done that from the beginning instead of waiting so long. It's a great way to hold yourself accountable and people are so encouraging. If I were starting my weight loss journey, I would definitely start posting on IG from day 1.

About May 19th I started feeling a bit tired and run down, sore from pushing myself during the workouts. For the first time since February I skipped a workout rather than push through. It broke my 3x weekly workout streak, but it's better to listen to your body.

For the rest of May I took it easy with the workouts, either skipping them or doing modified routines with lighter weights, not pushing myself. Besides, with all the packing and moving, I was lifting plenty of weights!

On the day we moved I weighed myself for the last time in that house: 143.0 – YES! Maintained, didn't gain!

May Status

- Starting Weight – 143.5
- Ending Weight – 143.0
- Pounds Lost – 0.5
- Total Lost – 79.5 lbs since Feb 1, 2016

Notes & Lessons Learned

- If I were starting my weight loss journey, I would definitely start posting on Instagram from DAY 1 – just do it!

June 2017

The first month living without my children was rough. I felt like a failure. Did I let them down by not trying harder to keep the family together?

I've said it before several times but it bears repeating – **weight loss is more mental than physical.**

Since February 2016 I'd been pretty focused on getting the weight off and getting myself together mentally. But kids grow up when you're not looking, and mine wanted to go out and try their wings. I understood but they were still my babies and I missed them terribly. So all of that was weighing heavily on my spirit.

Plus it's so damn hot in Texas! There was much to be done at the new place, and that kept me busy for the first few weeks of June. Getting settled, painting, hanging pictures, more purging.

It took 10 days before the TM was finally set up. I was too busy to drive to the park every day. That made it hard to hit my 10,000 steps, much less the 20,000 that I needed to maintain my way of eating. Yes I **love** to eat, and exercise is how I pay for it!

In the meantime, everybody in my family said I was getting too skinny. Harrianne, Theresa, Mark, even my kids said that's enough, don't lose anymore weight. Heh, they're all used to me being 200+ pounds so I guess 140 does look skinny to them.

On June 9th the TM was finally set up. Once again I was able to walk any time of day or night. The next day I jumped on the scale for the first time since May 31st and was shocked to see 141.5 - seriously??? That was a real surprise – I'd felt sluggish and fat, but instead had lost a couple pounds, only a couple away from the 130s!

Settling In

For the next 10 days I continued to sort, toss, and get organized. It was a struggle to get 10K steps in, much less 15-20K. What steps I did manage were all indoors, not the more strenuous outdoor steps. And still no strength training.

On June 19th I finally lifted weights for the first time in 3 weeks and it felt good! It took awhile, but I finally got back into the groove toward the end of the month.

All of that snacking and the stress of moving definitely took its toll. At the end of the month my weight was back up to 145.0, which I did NOT record in MFP.

June Status

- Starting Weight – 143.0
- Ending Weight – 145.0
- Difference – 2 lbs GAINED
- Total Lost – 77.5 lbs since Feb 1, 2016

Notes and Lessons Learned

- Summers are brutally hot in Texas, therefore I didn't walk outdoors as much, meaning less strenuous workouts.
- I cooked a lot more comfort food this month to keep us going while we moved and got settled – fried catfish, fries, enchiladas, teacakes, etc.
- I ate more dairy this month, which no doubt contributed to that

2 pound weight gain

- I bought a t-shirt that describes my philosophy perfectly: "I Work Out Because I Really Like Food"

July 2017

My starting weight was 145.0, so I gained 2 pounds in June – not exactly a surprise with all the crap I'd been eating. I missed living with my kids, and worried about them being out on their own. My ex-husband left the state for good, and I missed the emotional support he provided in dealing with the kids.

All of this plus moving and getting settled into a new place left me a bit drained. Not to mention the Houston heat, ugh. Not happy times.

Are you an emotional eater? I must confess, I am. In the month of July, this led to eating lots of fried food – catfish and fries, drum fish. Wine and cheese. Pizza and teacakes. I even had a hamburger. Any of this would be fine a little at a time, but all in one month was too much, hence the weight gain. I definitely felt heavier just from those couple extra pounds.

Again, it makes you wonder how on earth we allow ourselves to gain 20-30+ pounds without noticing, when our bodies are clearly giving us feedback all along the way. Truth is, we do see it but choose to ignore it. Denial...

Back to Basics

It took almost the whole month of July to get things back under control. Toward the end of the month, I finally went back to the basics – smoked tilapia and spinach, grilled chicken, etc. It felt good to eat healthy again. I also got back into the habit of walking in the evenings.

I attended my Aunt Julia's 101st birthday dinner in mid-July and got *lots* of questions from family members about my weight loss. Funny thing is, everybody wanted tips, but *nobody* wanted to hear "eat well, move a lot". No matter what, people seemed to think there was some elusive secret, a shortcut to a slim trim figure. If only that were true...

On July 17th I finally got back to weight training after a few weeks off. I had lifted weights only 3 times in the month of July, and my body really missed it.

The lack of strength training quickly showed up. I ended up gaining another 2.5 pounds, which put me back at my original 147.5 goal. I was still under 150 pounds and grateful for that. I had to get my ass back in gear – a birthday trip to Los Angeles was looming...

July Status
- Starting Weight – 145.0
- Ending Weight – 147.5
- Difference – 2.5 lbs GAINED
- Total Lost – 75 lbs since Feb 1, 2016

Notes & Lessons Learned
- I like being this size, and it looks like it takes 20k steps daily to stay this size and still eat the way I want. It's a good thing I like

walking.

- Maintenance sucks...

August 2017

August 1st marked 18 months since I began my weight loss journey on February 1, 2016. Since then I had gone from 222.5 to 147.5 – 75 pounds.

Yes, I faced the scale and it was not pretty – a 2.5 pound weight gain in July – OUCH! All those damn teacakes, along with the fried catfish, shrimp, bread, and everything but the kitchen sink. My exercise habit is what saved me.

Anyway, after a rough couple of months, it was now August, which meant that fall was around the corner, and the hot weather would finally fade away, eventually.

Summer has always been my **least** favorite time of year in Houston. It's the time when I'm most likely to gain weight because I get less outdoor exercise.

Was I upset? Hell no! I was "restarting" at 147.5, NOT 222.5, so all I felt was gratitude! I had enjoyed every lick, bite, and sip, but it was time to get back to the low 140s before my birthday trip to Los Angeles!

Back to Basics

I went back to eating healthy 80% of the time instead of the 60-40 split of the last couple months, when I ate badly more often than not.

Why I gained weight gain was no mystery – MFP always tells the story. Most days had ended in the red (calories over) instead of in the green (calories remaining). That always leads to weight gain!

So I cut back a little on fruit, which is high in carbs and sugar. I also reduced my dairy intake, and ate less yogurt bars and frozen yogurt, all those cool soothing foods that helped make the summer heat more bearable.

And finally I cut way back on teacakes, which was hard because I truly loved them. They're such a great comfort food. They even taste good cold!

I went back to my typical dinner – spinach/spring mix with salmon, tilapia or shrimp, or tuna with eggs. And lots of chopped salad.

Also I got back to strength training 3 times per week, sometimes doing a Jenny Ford routine. I was kinda weak on the lunges and push-ups, but other than that did pretty much everything. But I still reverted back to the Ashli workout when in a hurry or low on energy.

My weight finally started to come down in mid-August. By August 8th it was 145.5 – YES! Down, down, down it went.

I loved wearing tank tops for the first time in forever, and bought quite a few of them.

In late August Hurricane Harvey hit Houston **hard**. Fortunately we all weathered the storm just fine. We never lost power, so I was able to keep walking the entire time. After a few days Harvey finally left and we were none the worse for wear – very lucky!

August Status

- Starting Weight – 147.5

- Ending Weight – 143

- Pounds Lost – 4.5

- Total Lost – 79.5 lbs since Feb 1, 2016

Notes & Lessons Learned

- A small weight gain is no reason to panic, as long as you nip it in the bud right away. Get back on it and move forward from there.

September 2017

By September 1st I had lost the 4-1/2 pounds gained over the summer and was back down to 143.0 – YAY! The L.A. trip was only 19 days away so I had to be ON it!

My morning routine included "oil pulling", where you swish a tablespoon of coconut oil in your mouth for 20 minutes, followed by a mouthwash rinse. My friend Andrea had turned me onto this little trick for relieving tooth pain until you can get to a dentist. Anyway, a great side effect of this oral routine is that it killed my appetite, and made it easier to do intermittent fasting if desired.

I developed the habit of having a cup of grapes after the oil pull, walking for 1-2 hours, then strength training and smoothie. On non workout days, I would eat fruit, yogurt, or eggs for breakfast.

The weather finally started getting cooler so I went back to walking outdoors more. I was back to eating healthy and loving it. Teacakes became a rare treat instead of a daily indulgence.

I continued with the Ashli strength training workout and every now and then did a Jenny Ford routine.

On September 19th when I left for Los Angeles, my weight was 143.5 -- only 4 pounds from the 130s.

Back to Los Angeles

It was wonderful to be back in the City of Angels. My friend Linnette was in town, and we wasted no time getting out for some exercise. We went to Del Cerro park, the hiking trail I had discovered the previous summer.

We hiked several miles downhill and it was great – being 40 pounds lighter than last year, I could finally keep up with Linnette! When we got back to the top, Fitbit recorded that hike as 100 flights of stairs. I definitely posted *that* to the Fitbit hiking group and to Instagram! I was so tired I wasn't even hungry

A couple days later we hiked Kenny Hahn park, which we had done the previous summer. Again, it was so much fun to be able to keep up with Linnette, I actually gave her a run for her money. All those hills in LA are no joke! The only flat walks were at the beach, otherwise it was up and down hills all the time.

That evening I met my friend Marina for happy hour. When I arrived, she had ordered biscuits and sausage links. I ate a link but had NO desire to eat a biscuit. None. And I used to love nothing better than biscuits with butter and syrup. Who would have thought? Eat healthy long enough, and your body will soon reject everything else.

Beach Life

As usual I was staying at my friend Marci's place, near Palos Verdes. From there I roamed up and down the coast, hanging out with all my dearest friends. One day it was Andrea and Steven, who live in Manhattan Beach and lead a very vegan, very green lifestyle. Everything they eat is plant based and uber healthy. Not a fish or fowl in sight. It's become a running joke – every time I visit them, at some point we have to make a run to El Pollo Loco to get me some chicken!

Another day it was Redondo Beach with my friend Louie. We walked from Redondo Pier to Hermosa Pier and back. Then we found a shrimp lovers place on the boardwalk, yum. Earlier we had gone hiking in Del Cerro Park with Sherwin. So yeah, lots of hiking!

One day a group of us went to Venice Beach for a day of strolling and people watching. We stopped to have New York style pizza at one of my all-time favorite places. In years past, I had easily been able to eat 2 slices. But for some reason it didn't taste as good. All I could think about was how greasy it was and the number of carbs in each slice. I barely ate one slice. WTH? Is this what happens when you eat healthy? I guess your taste in food definitely changes and your body rejects stuff you used to really like. But still...

Here's a selfie taken on my last day being 61!

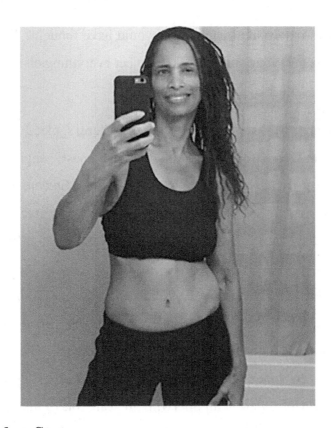

September Status

- Starting Weight – 143.0

- Ending Weight – ???

- Pounds Lost – ???

- Total Pounds Lost – 79.5+ lbs since Feb 1, 2016

Notes & Lessons Learned

- Anything is possible when you put your mind to it

October 2017

On October 1st I celebrated my 62nd birthday in Los Angeles with my closest friends, people I've known for 30+ years. It was one of my best birthdays ever.

Usually I weigh myself on the 1st day of the month. But every scale is different, so you should always use the same scale if you're tracking your weight. Well that scale was back in Houston so I didn't weigh myself, on this of all days...

For my birthday dinner, I met up with Andrea, Steven, Cheryl, Linnette, Kori, and Louie. We went to Tony Ps in Marina Del Rey and it was wonderful! Afterwards we walked around the Marina, so I got my 10k steps in, even on my birthday.

I spent the next few days chilling and relaxing. Visited with friends, walking on the beach, hanging out in Redondo Beach. It was so relaxing. And every day I walked at least 10k steps, usually in the sand.

There's something so invigorating about being in L.A., which is why I go back so often. Truth is, I feel more alive in California than anywhere else. All of the people who know me best live there. The climate, the hiking, it really is paradise. But my children are in Houston, which always draws me back.

October 6th was the perfect last day in L.A. We got sandwiches from Jersey Mike's, then went to Venice Beach. There we sat on the sand, ate, and people watched. The next day I headed back to Houston.

Back to Houston

After a couple days with the kids I finally got back to my scale on October 9th. My weight had been 143.5 when I left on September 19th. After 3 weeks in California I wasn't sure what to expect. So I was truly shocked when the scale said **137.5 – WHAT?** I could not believe it. I pulled the scale out to middle of the floor, weighed myself 4 or 5 times and it was 137.5 every time. WTF?

I had never imagined weighing 137.5 pounds *ever again in life*, so to be at that weight was unreal. And to lose 6 pounds while on vacation? I didn't know what to think. It must have been all that hiking!

Family members started to say stuff like, "It looks like you lost more weight", and "How much do you weigh now?" and "You've lost too much."

Well I didn't care what anybody said, I LOVED my new size, and decided I wouldn't mind getting down to 135. There was no reason to be concerned about an eating disorder – I love eating too much for that to happen. No, 135 was a nice pipe dream but at this point my biggest concern was to keep the weight off.

I still couldn't believe my weight was under 140, less than 10 pounds from my lowest adult weight *ever.* Now I just had figure out how to stay there...

Back to Weight Lifting

On October 16th I finally got back to strength training. It had been exactly one month since the last time, and the weights seemed to have gotten heavier in the interim.

In the meantime, the weather outside was glorious! I was finally able to walk outdoors on a regular basis again. I also did a couple of walks with a group called Girltrek.

Once again, I had to rein in my dairy consumption, which had definitely increased after I discovered and fell in love with Gorgonzola cheese in L.A.

Between the cheese and another round of teacakes, my weight crept up a bit, and I ended the month at 139.5. Still under 140 so not bad!

October Status

- Starting Weight – ????
- Ending Weight – 139.5
- Pounds Lost – ???
- Total Lost – 83 lbs since Feb 1, 2016

Notes & Lessons Learned

- Oil pulling works! I hadn't had a toothache in months but after only one week of not doing it, the tooth pain was back. Since then I've gotten dental work done, but still oil pull every day.
- While I was in L.A. my friend Cheryl introduced me to her niece Chanel (@BriskWalkLady on Instagram), who lost 90 pounds by walking. I encouraged her to start lifting weights. She encouraged me to start a podcast featuring people who've

lost weight, and offered to be my guest.

November 2017

On November 1ˢᵗ I was pleasantly surprised to see 139.5 on the scale, especially with the way I'd been eating since the L.A. trip. That put me at the 83 pound mark. It **HAD** to be the strength training – nothing else could explain still being in the 130s with the way I'd been eating.

For the first couple weeks of November I felt a bit under the weather with some upper respiratory allergy thing. This happened every time I ate more yogurt and cheese. You'd think that I would remember this when food shopping, but **NO**.

I resolved to cut out dairy completely, and started sipping ACV straight from the bottle. I also started using the Neti pot again.

Maintenance Adjustments

It was then that I realized that my custom eating program needed some adjustments. Maintenance is a whole different ballgame from losing. Something needed to replace the Gorgonzola cheese and yogurt bars. But not just any old calories – it needed to be the right mix.

Plus I wasn't eating enough in the mornings before walking and strength training, which is when my body needed some nourishment. Clearly those missing sugar and dairy calories need to be replaced with something. It's no wonder I was feeling run down and under the weather. And my water consumption was down.

I started eating more protein and drinking more water, and by mid-

November was feeling better. It was a constant struggle to eat enough of the right things, and not too much of the wrong things. I had to keep reminding myself that I was no longer trying to lose weight, that the goal was to stabilize.

Thanksgiving was different and bittersweet – the kids weren't around to help make the gumbo so I had to do it alone. I tasted it before the rice was ready and it was **so** good. So now I was eating gumbo without rice – how things had changed! We all got together on Thanksgiving Day, but still, I missed the good old days...

November Status

- Starting Weight – 139.5
- Ending Weight – 137.5
- Pounds Lost – 2
- Total Lost – 85 lbs since Feb 1, 2016

Notes & Lessons Learned

- It was definitely an adjustment giving up dairy, I missed having yogurt, yogurt bars and cheese.
- I tried Kind Bars, not sure if protein bars make good meal substitutes but they're ok for something quick.
- Tried KFC grilled wings and they were SO delicious, definitely must do again. Lots of protein and almost no carbs!
- Tried steel oats again, still not a fan.
- Near the end of the month I had a physical exam and the doctor

said not to lose too much weight. Too funny – I still had to get used to hearing that!

- I found a Jersey Mike's in my neighborhood and got the same sandwich we got in L.A. the Club Sub. It was even better than I remembered. Tons of carbs but still, so good. it definitely should be the ONLY meal of the day though!

December 2017

I got on the scale on December 1st – back to 137.5! YAY! Strength training continued to go well, still mostly the same Ashli routine from Gymbox.

Foodwise, I'd settled on some favorites that seemed to work well: grapes or whatever fruit is in season for breakfast, smoothies, sauteed tilapia and steamed spinach or salmon and broccoli or seafood gumbo or homemade chicken chili; pistachios for snacks, teacakes and pecan crowns for dessert.

Don't Let the Holidays Derail You

During the holiday season there are always parties and events just waiting to derail your eating plan. I learned to eat **before** going to any gathering, unless I was in charge of bringing one of the main dishes. That way I would know if there would be something good to eat and what was in it.

I had to keep reminding myself that I wasn't trying to lose weight, so no deficit was needed at the end of the day. But I didn't want to gain either so had to keep an eye on it.

This is the balancing game of the maintenance phase. It finally began to feel like second nature, or maybe I just got used to monitoring my intake vs output, and making sure they balance out. Skinny people do this all the time, but for former fatties, it's definitely a learned skill!

After weight training for 9 months, I'd finally started pushing myself to use heavier weights. Before that my inner child was like, "hey, be glad I'm doing it at all!". Eventually I felt stronger and wanted to get better, but that took a long time.

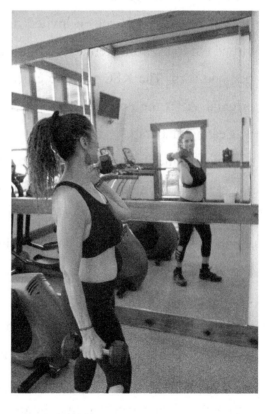

In mid December I took a peek at the scale and was shocked to see ... 133.0. Wow, when was the last time I saw THAT number?! I was truly shocked, but WTH???? Happy but still, 133.0?? Just 4 pounds away from the 120s. I could only attribute this to weight lifting.

If I had known how drastically strength training affects weight

loss, I would have started sooner!

On December 16th I went to lift weights with a friend at his community gym, and he really pushed me, hard.

I finally saw the value of a personal trainer or coach -- they'll push you *far* beyond what you'd do on your own. Because there is no way in hell I would have ever done what he made me do. I was SO tired afterwards, it was great!

The next day my cousin invited me to her place for lunch, which turned out to be from Kentucky Fried Chicken, plus some shrimp fried rice and corn. The KFC was the crispy fried kind, not grilled or even original. After the previous day's workout there was no way in hell I was eating that crap.

I picked the shrimp out of the rice. Didn't touch the corn. She tried to get me to eat more, saying, "Do it for me". I was like, "Nope, are you going to exercise it off for me?" Be prepared – people will try to sabotage your weight loss. I tore the skin off of one piece of chicken and ate that. I did have a glass of white zinfandel, that made her feel better.

After the mega workout on December 16th, I started doing the Ashli workout with 8 pounds where I would normally use 5 pounds. What a difference! I was winded and sweaty every time I finished. It was definitely a better workout than before. I could see muscles that were not there before, and thanked my guy friend for pushing me to the next level.

Toward the end of December I finally got so bored with the Ashli workout that I tried the Jenny Ford Classic weight training 50 minute workout. OMG. I discovered that I could do **real** push-ups and almost complete lunges! When did this happen?! It was a long workout, with lots of reps and I was ecstatic to get to the cool down.

Here's what I learned – your body is amazing and can do way more than you think. Ignore your lazy inner child and push yourself.

December Status

- Starting Weight – 137.5
- Ending Weight – 133.0
- Pounds Lost – 4.5
- Total Lost – 89.5 lbs since Feb 1, 2016

Notes & Lessons Learned

- I weighed 133.0 on January 1st 2018, exactly 20 pounds less than January 1st 2017! This was totally unexpected. I didn't set out to lose more weight, but that's the magic of weight lifting. It can be hard to get started, but the results are amazing.
- It pays to push yourself or find someone to do it for you.
- Always eat **before** going to any gathering unless you're bringing one of the main dishes. That way you know for sure there will be something good to eat and exactly what's in it. Constant vigilance is the name of the game!
- I tried the instant steel cut oaks and they didn't taste any worse

than the 30 minute version. In that sense they're an improvement, but I still don't like steel cut oats, so decided to regular oatmeal instead. It may not be as good for me, but if I don't like it, I'm not eating it. Life's too short to eat *anything* you don't like.

January 2018

Happy New Year! Jumped up, checked my weight and guess what – 133.0! I'm always shocked at a good weigh-in, probably because I'm not on a "diet" per se. I eat all my favorite foods and don't feel deprived.

My weight was down 89.5 pounds down since February 1, 2016. Just for fun and to make it an even 90 pounds, I decided to go for 132.5. But later for that...it was time to start the real battle – maintenance!

Who would have thought 2 years ago that I'd be able to lose 90 pounds? Here's the lesson: **just start.** I had no idea where this journey would lead. I wanted to weigh 148, and never imagined getting to 133.0. Who knew?

Usually at the first of the year I would make some weight loss resolution. Not this year. How amazing is that? No, this year my resolution was to **KEEP it off**!

Time to Get Off the Treadmill

Now it was time to work on other areas of my life. I resolved to get off the treadmill -- meaning get out of the house and back into the world. Time to figure out my "third act" of life!

On January 15th we marked the 3 year anniversary of our Mother's death. I met my sister Harri at the grave, we put fresh flowers all around and remembered the good times. We still wish she was here with us, but it definitely has become easier with time.

This is the end of the weight loss portion of my journey, mostly because there's nothing new to report. I eat quite a bit and walk a lot to pay for it. I eat healthy 80% of the time, and the other 20% have whatever I want. I've started intermittent fasting on a regular basis, and love the results.

This is how thin people eat except they don't talk about it. It's not remarkable because it's their lifestyle. And it's no longer remarkable for me because it's just how I eat. And exercise. And live.

January Goals

This month was full of a lot of introspection, as is often the case in the month of January. Now that I was finally fit, it was time to focus on other things while maintaining my weight loss.

Now it was time to get the rest of my life together. Pull myself out of the funk I had been in since my divorce and my mother's death. We're talking 4-5 years here, so this change was *way* overdue.

To be honest, that's why I focused on weight loss for the previous couple years – at least THAT was something I could control. Now I finally felt strong enough to point that resolve onto something else.

I continued to do the oil pulling, with amazing results. If you have tooth pain, try it! Swish 1 tablespoon of coconut oil around in your mouth for 20 minutes, then rinse with a couple capfuls of non-alcoholic mouthwash. It works! (Then get thee to a dentist, ASAP ...)

I settled into a morning routine that works – oil pull, rinse, cup of grapes, walk for a bit, then strength training 3 times a week. Followed by a smoothie. If no strength training, then walk while working or whatever at the treadmill desk, run errands, hang out with the kids, etc. Really there's nothing left to say about it. It's a lifestyle now. Sometimes I don't eat enough, other times too much. That's maintenance. That's life! Works for me. What works for you?

Full Circle Moments

January 24th marked the 3 year anniversary of Mom's funeral. What a full circle moment. On that day in 2015 I watched Mom being lowered into the ground. I weighed over 200 pounds and felt absolutely miserable.

One year later (2016) I weighed 220+ pounds, felt "the click" and decided to change my life.

A year later (2017) I'd lost 75 pounds.

And on this day 3 years later (2018), I weighed 132.5 pounds.

Status

- Starting Weight – 133.0
- Ending Weight – 132.5
- Pounds Lost – 0.5
- **Total Lost – 90 lbs since Feb 1, 2016**

Notes & Lessons Learned

- February 1, 2018 - 132.5 lbs!

- On January 9th my sister Harri and I visited our mother's grave on what would have been her 100th birthday. Harri gave me a zucchini bread loaf. I checked the label – 40g carbs per serving with 2-1/2 servings or 100 carbs in that little loaf! Read the labels!

- My new favorite kitchen appliance became the air fryer. It's great for getting a crispy crunchy texture without frying. Jillian Michaels mentioned it as hot trend.

- Went shopping for some new workout pants and had to buy size 4-6. They turned out to be too loose because there was no way to make them tighter in the waist so I ended up returning them. Amazing.

- I donated blood mid-month and felt a bit low energy for a couple days afterwards, but it's worth it to save lives. Years ago, I was told by the Red Cross that there's something about my blood that makes it good for premature babies, that they can divide my donation into 3 or 4 little bags and save that many babies. I dunno, but it has inspired me to keep giving ever since. And every couple months they send an email reminding me to donate.

- I had lost 90 pounds in 2 years and felt like I could accomplish anything. So can you. *See it. Believe it. Achieve it.*

- Never give up.

Maintenance

Beginning February 2018 my focus shifted from losing weight to the hardest part ... **maintenance.**

I had lost 90 pounds in 2 years. Nice, but I knew better than to relax and think the war was over. In reality, it had only just begun. If the past was any indication of success, it would be short lived. Let's review...

- In 1987 I had lost 45 pounds and got down to 129 lbs ... for about 5 minutes.

- Over the years I had lost and gained the same 20-30 pounds multiple times, for one reason or another – reunions, special occasions, whatever.

- In 2006-2007 I had lost 50 pounds after discovering the treadmill desk.

None of those losses were permanent because I had the temporary "diet" mindset. And I hadn't yet learned the importance of **consistently tracking and monitoring caloric input and output**.

What would be the plan going forward to make sure I didn't repeat the mistakes of the past?

The Slippery Slope

I recognized the need to continue to push myself, to try other strength training routines, maybe actually go to a gym, get a personal trainer, try yoga, etc. But honestly I was happy to have reached a steady state and just **wanted to maintain it.**

This is the slippery slope that derails most weight loss stories. Because of the "diet" mentality, we have a tendency to go on diets, then go off when we get "there".

This has to change if you're going to maintain weight loss long term. It's the paradigm shift, the big **CLICK**. I finally got it this time. There is no "there" and you're done. It's a hard truth to face but it's the *only* way to long lasting results.

Let's look at the definition of maintenance:

> *Maintenance* - " *the process of maintaining or preserving someone or something, or the state of being maintained. The upkeep of property or equipment.* "

Houses and cars need to be maintained. Your weight is no different. Especially if you had to work like hell to get it off.

Maybe it didn't require any effort when you were younger, but if you've had to WORK to get it off, you're going to have to KEEP WORKING if you want to keep it off. Maybe not as hard and as long, but still. Work. If you don't want to do this, don't bother to lose weight because ultimately it will find you again.

This is why so many people say it's harder to keep weight off than it is to lose it. Weight loss induced euphoria eventually wears off. Your new body becomes the norm, the novelty of being thin wears off, and you're left with … maintenance.

It had taken a long time and a lot of hard work to get my body to a normal weight. I knew from bitter experience that it would take constant vigilance, self-awareness and a healthy lifestyle to maintain it.

Lifestyle Rules

Knowing that eternal vigilance is the key to keeping the weight off, these are the "lifestyle" rules I've developed:

- Weigh myself at least once a week, and always on the first day of the month, just to be sure things are still on track.

- If not within 2 pounds of my desired weight, take action **immediately,** nip it in the bud, don't let it go any higher. Cut back on calories and up the exercise til those pounds are gone.

- Only eat food that I *love* and truly enjoy. This is non-negotiable. Life is too short to eat anything you don't like, even if it's more healthy for you. That's why I still eat white french bread ... with butter. Just not too much of it.

- Continue food logging with MFP and exercise tracking with Fitbit. Religiously. No need to obsess about carbs, just try to keep them under 150 per day, or closer to 100 if a bit fluffy and need to pull back...

- Continue to strength train 3 times a week, gradually increase weights, reps, etc. Push myself to try other types of workouts.

- Other than that, there are no rules – eat sensibly following the 80/20 rule and enjoy life.

PART III:

YOUR STEPS TO SUCCESS

Now it's your turn. There is only ONE perfect weight loss plan for you, and it's my belief that you won't find it in *any* off the shelf book or commercial weight loss program. Not unless you wrote it. It's time for *you* to create **your own** ideal food and exercise program, one that you can follow indefinitely.

There is no one size fits all or even most. There is **one** ideal way of eating *for you* that will allow you to lose weight while still enjoying your life. Your ideal program is customized *for you*. It's based on **your** life – your likes, dislikes, can't stands, must haves.

Truth is, you can lose weight on **any** diet. But if you want to *keep it off*, it has to be in a way that you can maintain for life. Cookie cutter food plans rarely work for long. Find what works for you — it's the only thing that will work long term.

If you can do that with one of the diets out there, more power to you. No commercial diet has ever worked long-term for me, so I can't endorse any of them.

Your job is to figure out what works for you – the food plan and exercise program that you can happily follow for the rest of your life.

What are you willing to give up? What's *non-negotiable*?

Before we get started, let's review some basics.

Step #1: Understand Weight Loss Basics

Everything you could possibly want to know about weight loss is freely available to you on the Internet, so there's no need to give you chapter and verse. A brief review of the basics so we're on the same page should suffice. Let's start with BMI.

What's Your BMI?

For years, the best way to know whether your weight was in a healthy range was to check it against those weight charts provided by the government. You can still find them online.

Today the medical community uses another standard for determining healthy weight, the **Body Mass Index (BMI).** It's not always totally accurate, but it's a quick and easy way to determine whether your body type would be classified as underweight, normal, overweight or obese.

Here's the BMI calculation formula for adults:

BMI = weight in pounds x 703 / height in inches^2

Or simply search Google for BMI Calculator, and you'll get a page full of them to try, including special calculations for teens and children.

For example:

Weight: 222.5 lbs (this is where I started!)

Height: 5'6" or 66 inches

BMI = (225.5 * 703) / 4356 = 35.9

This person has a BMI of **35.9** and considered Very Obese **(that was me!)**

Body Mass Index (BMI) Categories

- **Underweight**: BMI is less than **18.5**

- **Normal weight**: BMI is **18.5 to 24.9**

- **Overweight:** BMI is **25 to 29.9**

- **Obese**: BMI is **30 or more**

- **Very Obese**: BMI is **35 or more**

Another useful measuring tool is the **Basal Metabolic Rate (BMR),** which is different for every person. Your BMR is an estimate of how many calories you'd burn if you were to do nothing but rest for 24 hours. It represents the minimum amount of energy needed to keep your body functioning, including breathing and keeping your heart beating.

I haven't thought about BMR *even once* during this entire weight loss journey, so I can't speak about it. But if you want more info, search the web for BMR calculators. Some BMI calculators include BMR calculations as well.

Calories 101

You hear the word "calories" a lot, as in something to avoid if you want to lose weight. In reality, a calorie is simply a measurement of energy, which is produced by the food you eat when it's burned by your body.

Every human needs calories to keep their body going. The average human needs 2,000 calories per day. This can be more for larger people and athletes, and less for smaller people and children.

If you eat 2,000 calories every day and burn 2,000 calories every day, the balance remains the same, i.e. you don't gain weight.

However, if you eat 2,500 calories and your body only burns 2,000, those 500 extra calories will be stored as fat. It usually happens gradually.

You might not even notice it immediately, but your body will keep track of every calorie. Repeat this 7 times and you've gained a pound. Eventually 1 pound becomes 5, then 10, and you know the rest. The more excess calories you eat, the faster your fat stores grow.

In order to reverse this trend, you must burn off more calories than you consume. The more calories you burn off, the less fat stores you'll have. This also happens gradually – and spending fat is definitely not as much fun as spending money!

Bottom line: Your body stores fat in order to have access to energy whenever it needs it. When you eat more than your body needs, it shows up as fat. In this case, a higher "bank" balance is not a good thing.

Well, it would be great in case of a famine – you'd outlive all the skinny people around you. But barring that, you have way more potential energy than the body needs. That's all that fat is really – potential energy.

Calories Do Count

Weight loss is simple. Not easy, but simple. There are 3,500 calories in every pound. Your body needs a certain number of calories to sustain itself. When you take in more than your body needs, extra weight is the result.

To lose weight, you need to consume less than the body needs so that it will use the fat stored on your body to make up the deficit. Unfortunately there are no shortcuts. You can't beat the math.

Speaking of math, what is about that subject that strikes fear into our hearts? I didn't want to count calories either, and looked for every way possible to avoid it.

But once you get started, it quickly becomes automatic. We all tend to eat the same foods over and over, and you'll soon learn the calorie counts of all your favorites. If you use a tool like MFP, it will do most of the work for you.

Counting calories is really not that bad. You must be honest with yourself and stay vigilant, but once you get the hang of it, calorie counting becomes second nature. It's something that you do for yourself, and your life will be better because of it.

How Many Calories Are In a Pound?

There are 3,500 calories worth of energy in a pound of fat. Weight loss is a simple formula: burn more calories than you consume.

To lose one pound of fat per week, you need to burn 3,500 calories more than you consume. There are 3 ways you can achieve this:

- eat 500 calories *fewer* every day

- burn off an *extra* 500 calories every day

- a *combination of the two* – eat less, move more

While it's possible to lose weight solely by reducing calories, most health professionals will agree that losing weight via diet *and* exercise is far better. I definitely find it far easier to combine the two – give up some calories while burning off even more.

For example, say your body needs 2,000 calories per day to survive. You go for a walk, or hop on the treadmill for a couple hours while checking your email, reading a book, looking at TV or talking on the phone. At the end of the day your body would have used up 2,500 calories – the 2,000 you'd normally burn off, plus the 500 from the exercise.

Now, instead of eating the 2,000 calories you'd normally consume, you cut back and eat only 1,500 calories. You've just created a 1,000 calorie deficit – 500 from eating less, 500 from exercise. That's an extra 1,000 calories that your body has to get from somewhere. Where's that? All of that fat hanging around your waist, butt, and thighs, that's where! Keep this up for 7 days and you've lost 2 pounds.

It's just that simple.

Or eat the whole 2,000 calories per day while continuing to walk off 500 calories and you'll only lose 1 pound. It's a slower pace, but better than nothing. And 2,000 calories a day is a LOT of food – that's what I eat on my "whatever I want" days!

I look at this as a game: how much **enjoyment** and **nourishment** I can get out of calories consumed vs. how much exercise I have to do to earn them. Maybe it won't work for you, but it's how I've been able to trick my body into losing 90 pounds.

Does it always work? Will it always result in losing 2 pounds a week. No. **Weight loss is *not linear.* ** Many factors affect your weight loss/gain during the week, but over time, it all evens out. You might lose 2 pounds this week, zero next week, and 4 pounds the week after that. Stay the course, trust the process, and the scale will steadily march downward.

Maintain a Caloric Deficit

To lose weight, *calories expended has to be greater than calories consumed.* Once I finally got this, it became a game of maintaining a caloric deficit.

Throughout the day, keep a running tab on your remaining calories

— at the end of the day that number should be 1,000 if you want to lose 2 pounds a week.

While it is possible to lose weight through diet alone, it's a long hard road. And you'll be hungry a lot. In my mind, exercise is a must. Even a little is better than nothing.

Some days I walk quite a bit and end up with a big calorie deficit. This is like found money! I can save it, meaning I'll lose weight a bit faster. Or I can have a snack – maybe a handful of nuts, a yogurt bar, or a cookie. Or even a piece of cake.

Now, maybe I don't have a big deficit and still want the piece of cake. Do I get back on the TM and earn it? Or take my lumps and end the day in the red on MFP?

It's a game, remember that. This works for me. It really makes me think, how bad do I want that piece of cake. Enough to walk another 2 hours? Usually not, but at least it's a conscious choice.

This is how I was able to indulge so much when I was going through the teacake phase. I loved them so much that it was worth it to walk a couple hours while watching a football game, just to satisfy that craving.

A lot of times, whatever it is you want ends up not tasting that good, but the craving is gone, you don't feel deprived, and you'll have no trouble resisting it the next time.

When you eat this way, it all becomes a game you play with yourself. It's a way of keeping your inner child happy while the adult you works toward your fitness goals.

That's really it. Remember – consistency over time equals results. Trust the process and just do it.

Do You Really Lose a Pound of Fat for Every 3,500 Calories You Burn?

I read an article titled, "You Need to Burn 7,000 Calories to Lose a Pound, Not 3,500". It claims that most overweight people will lose about half the weight that the 3,500-calories rule predicts, so that the new rule is 7,000 calories = one pound. Blah, blah, blah. Google it if you're interested.

Well, what they're saying is what I've said all along – weight loss is not linear and that it comes off over time, in fits and starts. But to say that 3,500 doesn't equal a pound is ridiculous.

Yes, the body needs fewer calories as your weight reduces, but as long as you're using a tool that takes this into account like MFP, and continue to maintain a 500-1000 calorie a day deficit, you'll continue to lose weight. And 3,500 calories does indeed equal a pound!

Anyway, it doesn't matter. As long as you're eating and exercising in a way that's delightful and satisfying, it doesn't matter how long it takes.

Remember, this is a *lifestyle*, not a diet that you go on (and off). It's not a sprint, it's a marathon, one that *will never end*. As long as you're not deprived, it really doesn't matter how long it takes. And you'll have a much better chance of maintaining your weight loss once you reach goal. Frankly, the slower you lose, the better chance you have of keeping it off.

Some Tips...

- Aim to lose 1-2 pounds a week while fully enjoying your life, not feeling deprived.

- Find a mindless exercise that you enjoy – walking, biking, swimming, any activity you like and will do consistently.

- Exercise more instead of cutting out calories. It's not that hard, just move your ass...

- Walk or move whenever possible – the more you do it, the more your body will love it; every step counts (research Dr. James Levine and NEAT).

- Consume about 30% protein, 40% carbs, and 30% fats.

- Don't deprive yourself of anything you like – plan for it ahead of time and account for it in your food logging.

You'll Need Some Tools

Here are a few things that will come in handy:

- Bathroom scale (preferably digital)

- Kitchen scale

- Set of measuring cups and spoons

- Blender for making smoothies

- Spiralizer

- Electric tea kettle

- A good pair of walking shoes

- Workout clothes

Ok, now that we've gotten the basics out of the way, let's move on to your actual steps to success.

Step #2: Know Your Why

Why do you want to lose weight? No, really... why? To look better, feel better, live longer, attract a mate, get a job, be around for your children? **Why?**

You've probably lost and gained hundreds of pounds over the years. I certainly had before 2016. What will be different this time? What will make it all "click" for you? How bad do you want it? And what are you willing to give up to get it?

As I've said over and over, **weight loss is more mental than physical.** Without the right mindset, you're wasting your time. Don't even bother starting, because you'll end up right where you started, with all the weight you lost and then some. Save yourself the deprivation and aggravation until you're ready. *Really* ready.

It's up to you to decide whether you've experienced "the click" and are ready to change your lifestyle.

In my case I was sick and tired of being **sick and tired**.

Sick of starting but never quite getting to a normal weight and staying there.

Tired of looking in the mirror and seeing an unhappy 200+ pound woman staring back, one who had to buy men's size 2XL shirts to cover her rather large ass.

Sick of not feeling sexy or attractive. Cute clothes are hard to find in size 20+.

Tired of knee aches, back aches and every kind of ache your body suffers from carrying around 90 extra pounds.

Sick of not wanting to get dressed up and go out because of having nothing to wear.

Tired of lugging around the equivalent of another person, 24 hours a day. And knowing that time was ticking by, relentlessly. Every day.

What's Your Motivation?

My mother was the liveliest person I knew, even in her 90s. Five days before her death, at her 97th birthday party, she talked about getting back on Facebook, and asked about her favorite football players. She's the reason I love football. This was on January 10th.

Fourteen days later, on January 24th, she was being lowered into the ground. That brought it home for me. The time is *now*. Do it **NOW** while you still can.

But it still took another whole year before I was really ready to do it...

What's your driving motivation to *really* lose weight this time and *keep it off*, no matter how many times you've failed in the past? That's "the click".

You start wherever you are – whatever your weight, it's going downward from there. That **has** to be your mindset. KNOW IT. SEE IT. BELIEVE IT. Otherwise, don't bother. Come back when you're clear on that.

What's your why? Write down all the reasons you hate being

obese. Be honest. Regardless of anything you might read about body acceptance and being fat positive, being overweight is a serious threat to your health. It's not *if* but *when* it will catch up with you.

Once you face up to this and decide to change your life no matter what, *this* is "the click". It's your new mindset, which you'll use to reach your goal this time. Even if you've never been able to do it before.

Commitment Outlasts Willpower

People sometimes ask about willpower, as in how do you find and keep it long enough to lose 90 pounds? It's not about willpower. It's about being committed to the lifestyle change that you have decided to make. It's about having a clear vision of your future, of your body at a normal weight. If you're doing something you really care about, you don't need willpower. The vision pulls you forward.

Do you need willpower to keep your body clean, comb your hair, take care of your family? No. It's just something that you do. Losing weight is no different. You have a plan and stick to it no matter what. It's not something you have to think about or choose to do. Commit to yourself. Then stay true to your commitment.

Once You Reach Goal

It's exciting to see pounds melting away, but at some point you will reach your goal. Then what? Once you've lost the weight, what will be your motivation to keep it off?

Now is the time to think about your vision for your new thin life. Make a list of everything you plan to gain from losing weight. What will your life be like then?

In my case, I already had a vision – the girl on the fence from 1987.

Yes I knew it wouldn't be exactly the same since I'm twice her age, but it gave me something to shoot for. I wanted to look good in clothes, and not have to shop in the plus size section to find them. I was determined to feel sexy again. To have more energy. To feel good about myself.

What's your vision? Write it down. Make a vision board. Get ready, because you will get there, and your mindset has to match your new body.

Chances are you'll learn a lot about yourself during your weight loss journey. That you're stronger than you thought. That you can do things you never imagined you could do.

And out of that you will learn to set new goals for yourself, have a desire to experience new things, and do whatever it takes to maintain your healthy new lifestyle.

Get ready...

Step #3: Set Your Goals

Ok, your mindset is right. You've experienced "the click" and you're really, *really* ready to do this.

You've figured out the right weight range for your age, sex and height.

Based on that and *your personal preference*, what is the right weight for you? The weight charts and BMI calculations give you a range, but it's up to you to decide what you want to weigh. Maybe you're not sure at first – choose a range.

Goals can change as you get closer to the ideal you, especially if you throw in some weight training. I initially chose 148 as my ideal weight, and never imagined that 131 to 136 would ever be MY weight range! Are you serious?

Start down the road and see where it leads you...just start.

Put It In Writing

A goal is **specific** and **measurable**. With a time limit. **In writing.**

"I want to lose some weight" or "I need to fit into this dress" – these are **not goals.**

Here's a goal: "I want to lose 60 pounds in one year, starting next week", or "I want to have a BMI of 24.9 by my 51st birthday, which means I need to lose 69 pounds".

Whatever it is, it has to be concrete. Something **definite,** with a time limit. Even if it ends up taking a bit longer to reach, it's still good to have a date attached to your goal.

Be Realistic

Your goal must be reasonable. Don't set yourself up for failure by saying you want to lose 100 pounds in 3 months. It's not going to happen. Not in a healthy way.

This is not a sprint. It's a marathon that will never end. Slow and steady is the way to go.

Remember, this going to be your *lifestyle*. **For life**. So it really doesn't matter how long it takes because you're not quitting when you get there, and you want to enjoy yourself along the way.

Wouldn't you rather lose "only" one pound a week in a way that doesn't feel like work, where you never feel deprived?

Or would you rather lose weight fast, be miserable along the way, and gain it all back when it's over? I've done both. Slower is better.

Having said all that, now it's time to set some realistic goals for yourself.

- What's your ideal weight? You can use weight charts as a guide, but only you can decide the best weight for your body. I'm 5'6" and decided I wanted to weigh under 150 pounds, so initially chose 148 as my goal to give myself some wiggle room. Strength training redefined my body and 135 became my new target weight.

- What's the right weight *for your body?*

- How much do you want to lose?

Go ahead, write down your goals. And mean them.

This is a binding agreement, a promise that you make to yourself. You may lie to someone else, but hopefully you don't lie to yourself.

Don't let yourself down.

Take Status Photos

Take pictures of yourself before and during your weight loss journey, no matter how painful. Full body pictures.

As I mentioned before, for some reason many of my initial "before" pics were just of my body, not showing my face. I was pretty new at taking selfies, maybe that was it. Deep down, I think it was my way of dissociating myself with the fat girl in the mirror.

Anyway, take photos frequently, you'll be amazed later on when you look back. Try to take them in the same place, pose, clothes, etc. You'll need those pictures when telling your own weight loss story.

Take Body Measurements

In addition to measuring the pounds on the scale, don't forget your body measurements. They can be even more telling.

As you lose fat you could be gaining muscle (especially if you add resistance training), but you won't know that just from looking at the numbers on the scale. That's only part of it. Routinely take your measurements as well.

Periodically Reassess

Your fitness and nutrition journey probably won't follow a straight line. As you lose weight, your goals might change.

In a long-term strategy, it's not just about food. It's about your life, and how your goals fit into it. Every once in awhile, life has a way of disrupting even the best laid plans.

Things happen. Your living situation may change. Your finances may get out of whack. You may reach your goal and look too skinny. These are all things that may prompt you to reassess your current fitness and nutrition strategy. Do your initial goals still make sense given your new situation?

In my case, because of the strength training, I surpassed my initial 74.5 pound goal and lost an additional 15.5 pounds. I didn't set out to lose 90 pounds, yet here I am. For the most part I'm able to maintain it, although during the summer my weight tends to go up a bit. As long as it's in the vicinity of 135, I'm happy. I'm not a slave to healthy eating, nor to a specific number on the scale.

Remember, you make the rules for your life. And you can rewrite them any time you please. It's all about what works for you. And what works for you – like life – can change over time. Or in the blink of an eye...

Step #4: Make Your Food Plan

You know what you want to weigh.

You know that this is a lifestyle you're embarking upon. Not a diet that you're going to go on, then off. This is *for life*.

To that end, plan on losing 1-2 pounds a week until you get to your goal. Some weeks it may be less, or even more, but that's a realistic target to aim for. It's totally doable if you **stay conscious** and **hold yourself accountable**.

Ready? Let's get started.

Follow a Diet or Create Your Own?

The first decision you have to make is, are you going to follow a "diet" or create your own plan. You know how I feel about diets, but perhaps you need the structure of being told what to eat, when to eat, and how much to eat.

As long as it's not so restrictive that you can't enjoy your life, that's fine. Remember, you have to eat this way *for the rest of your life*, or at least a modified version once you reach your goal. Otherwise the weight will come back.

There are programs out there that give a wide range of foods to choose from and remove the need to count or track calories.

Some programs even offer pre-packaged meals so you don't have to do the math or the cooking. They may disguise the measurements as points, units, exchanges or whatever. It still boils down to calories, just like ALL weight loss programs. There's no escaping it because that's the energy system that *every* human body uses. **Calories**.

But hey, whatever works for you. If that's a commercial diet, great. Since I don't endorse or promote any particular eating program, it doesn't matter to me.

My only concern is that you find a healthy way of eating **that you can follow for life.** My eating program is solely based on foods I truly enjoy, and is included only as a point of reference, not to suggest that anyone should eat that way.

Things to Consider

Whether you choose a diet or create your own, you need to **make a plan** for how you're going to lose weight and keep it off. Here are some things to consider when deciding:

- Is it healthy? <u>No</u> food groups should be off limits, including carbs and fats. It all belongs.

- Is it flexible enough to fit your lifestyle? Some people have specific cultural or ethnic requirements when it comes to food.

- Think about your experience with past diets. What have you tried before? What worked or didn't work for you? Were you able to follow the diet? How did you feel while on the diet, both physically and emotionally?

- Do you have health issues that need to be considered, such as allergies, diabetes, heart disease, etc? Consult your doctor before starting, just to be safe.

- Do you like to diet on your own, or do you need support such as from a group? If you want group support, do you prefer online support or face to face meetings?

- Some commercial weight loss programs require you to buy meals or supplements. For people who don't want to be bothered with cooking, one of these programs might be ideal because it removes the fuss and bother of cooking and measuring. Others might require in person visits to weight loss clinics or support meetings. Do these things fit into your budget?

- You need a plan to lose weight, but it doesn't have to be complicated. A few simple rules will do. Your job is to figure out what will work for *you* – what food and exercise plan you can happily follow *for the rest of your life?*

Food Logging Works

Whether you decide to follow a commercial diet or create your own, I truly believe that food logging – keeping a "diet diary" – is critical for weight loss success.

I've lost and gained *many* pounds over the years, and all of the weight gains happened when I was not actively food logging. I can't explain it. I only know that **FOOD LOGGING WORKS.**

Since Feb 1st 2016, I've religiously recorded every bite, lick, and sip into **MyFitnessPal**. Everything. If I don't know the exact nutritional info, it's easy to find something similar in the huge database of foods and record that. Some MFP notes:

- Initially my daily calorie target was 1550, based on my weight and how quickly I wanted to lose weight. I chose 2 pounds a week, which is a calorie deficit of 1000 calories a day. That's actually a lot of calories to give up, which is why it's hard to lose more than 2 pounds a week in a healthy way without exercise. Who wants to live on less than 1,000 calories per day?

- As you lose weight, your body will need fewer calories to sustain itself, so your daily calorie target will decrease, otherwise you'll stop losing. My daily target is now 1290. But because I exercise so much, I can eat up to 1800 calories per day and not gain weight.

I use MFP because it's free, easy to use, and has a gigantic database of every possible food known to man, including all the top fast food places. You can even input your own recipes. It's amazing. Did I mention it's free?

By the way, if MFP is not your cup of tea, there are many other calorie counting and food tracking tools to choose from – a quick Google search will give you a long list.

Getting Started With MyFitnessPal

If you decide to try MFP, simply download and install it on your phone. It also works on tablets and your desktop.

Once you create an account, you need to complete your profile and enter your goal weight. MFP will then tell you the maximum number of calories per day you should eat to achieve that goal.

The paid version of MFP gives you more information about macro-nutrients but after all this time I still use the free version.

The default MFP recommendation is to consume 20% protein, 50% carbs and 30% fat. There are online calculators that can help you figure out your ideal macro intake. I wouldn't worry too much about the exact numbers as long as calories are on track and you're eating healthy most of the time.

Track everything you eat or drink. **Everything**. Even if you're not tracking calories per se, there's something about seeing everything you consume recorded somewhere that holds you accountable in ways you can't imagine. Just do it. You'll be amazed.

Create Your Own Food Plan

First of all, you have to clearly identify all the foods in your life that you absolutely love and can't imagine not being able to have. Write them down.

Based on your likes, dislikes, must haves and can't stands, you'll create a way of life that you can live with... forever.

Here are some guidelines:

- Make a list of all your favorite foods, whatever they are.

- Focus on whole foods as much as possible (lean proteins, fruit, veggies, legumes, etc.).

- Focus on more fruits, vegetables, nuts, seafood, high quality oils, lean meats, quality dairy and whole grains.

- Eat the highest quality calories that you can, i.e. delicious satisfying food made with fewer calories.

- Make meals from scratch whenever possible. The more you cook for yourself, the better off you'll be. At least you'll know exactly what you're eating. If your lifestyle doesn't allow time for cooking, there are some great pre-packaged fresh meals available that are healthy and satisfying ... but these can be pricey.

- No food group should be off limits. Carbs, fats, proteins – they're all good and you need them ALL.

Plan Your Meals

Once you decide to create your own meal plan, you need to decide exactly what you're going to eat. The time to think about that is before you go to the grocery store. Make a list *before* you go shopping. And whatever you do, don't go food shopping when you're hungry!

Meal planning doesn't have to be complicated. Actually the simpler the better. Just come up with some healthy meal favorites and stick to them at first. When you get bored, create some new favorites and add them to the mix. Make it fun. Food should be fun.

Since this is *your* custom meal plan, I can't tell you what should be on it. But I will tell you what I eat, and give you some general guidelines.

Honestly you can find everything you need to know about nutrition online for free. It's not rocket science, just try to stick to the macro breakdown recommendation of 10-35% protein, 45-65% carbs, and 20-35% fats. That's a pretty wide range, so you should be able to find what works for you pretty easily. I aim for 30% protein, 40% carbs and 30% healthy fats.

If you look closely at the most popular diets, they're really not that different. Except for the extreme diets (ahem, cabbage soup), most of them emphasize the need to replace processed junk food with high quality, nutrient-dense, *whole foods*. These foods often contain fiber, will keep you satisfied longer and enable you to control your food intake.

Rather than being stuck in any one diet "box", develop an understanding of your body and works best for you, then create your nutritional strategy based on that.

At the Grocery Store

First of all, make a list. Shop from that list. And again, don't go food shopping on an empty stomach. Ever.

I remember reading somewhere that we should shop the outer edges of the store, meaning the produce, fresh and frozen food aisles. Anything that can sit on a shelf unrefrigerated usually contains preservatives with unpronounceable names. Think about that whenever you venture to the inside aisles.

Years ago a friend told me some of the things his brother used to tell him about working in a canning goods plant. I never forgot the stories he told me about the disgusting things the workers did to the food in vats during the canning process. Well, hopefully quality control has improved since then, but those stories made me rethink canned goods, and it's probably why I avoid most of them to this day.

Read Nutrition Labels

All packaged foods in the USA come with a nutrition label that includes the list of ingredients. Always read this list carefully. This is the only way to understand what's in the food you eat, and make healthier food choices.

Many nutrition labels are traps, designed to sucker you into thinking something is healthy when it's not. Do not let terms such as "light/lite", "fat free", "low calorie", "low fat", "zero trans fat" trick you into buying foods that are not nutritious.

A few label reading tips:

- Start at the top with serving size per container. If it's more than 1 serving, watch out! You need to multiply that times the calories per serving if you plan to eat the whole thing.

- Avoid trans fat. Be careful – if a food has less than 0.5 grams of trans fat per serving, the label can still read 0 grams trans fat. Check the ingredient list for partially hydrogenated vegetable oil, which indicates that some trans fat is included in the food, even if the amount is below 0.5 grams.

- Choose monounsaturated fats – these are the good fats found in olive oil, avocados and nuts.

- Try not to eat anything that contains more than 5 ingredients or ingredients that you can't pronounce.

- Avoid foods that contain preservatives and can be left on supermarket shelves indefinitely.

- Here's a nutrition label that shows the main things you should look for when comparing products. Visit the FDA website for more insight into understanding labels.

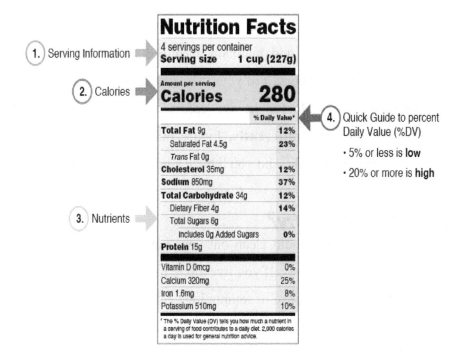

If Cooking Is Not For You...

Maybe you don't have time to cook every day. I read a weight loss memoir about a woman who didn't want to be bothered with cooking. Nor did she like vegetables. She decided to lose weight by calorie counting, and used all of her calories on fast food. And she refused to eat vegetables. Eventually she began to eat better, but at first this is what she did, and it worked for her.

Granted, those kind of meals aren't the best nutrition wise, but as long as you know that there's nothing off limits, it will hopefully help you make better choices going forward.

Fact is, you can lose weight by eating anything, as long as you account for the calories and maintain a caloric deficit. There is no reason to ever deprive yourself of your favorite foods.

Remember, **it's calories in vs. calories out, and don't let anybody tell you any differently.** Figure out what works for you, what fits into your lifestyle, and you'll have a better chance of success.

Clean Out Your Pantry?

I've read that you should clean out your pantry before embarking on your weight loss journey. If you live alone maybe that will work for you, but clearing your house of temptations can be challenging if you live with your family, and especially if you have young children.

The key is to keep healthy food and snacks on hand to make it easier to avoid temptation. It's a lot easier to resist unfriendly foods if you have a healthy alternative to grab instead. If you want to keep snacks around for your kids, try to choose things they they like, but that you *do not* like. Make it easy on yourself.

Actually, the more healthy food choices there are in the house, the more kids get used to eating that way. Most kids eat way too much processed food and junk anyway, which is why childhood obesity is on the rise. So perhaps cleaning out the pantry is not a bad idea. Just realize that it could meet with some resistance from other family members.

In my case, everybody in the house was grown, so that wasn't an issue for me. I simply didn't buy anything that I didn't plan to eat. My kids were old enough to buy their own snacks and hide them from each other, so I didn't have to worry about seeing any of it.

Here's What I Eat

As you know by now, I do **NOT** follow any particular diet or plan. That doesn't work for me. Over time I've come to truly enjoy and prefer healthy fare, but *nothing* is off limits. Ever.

For the most part, I tend to eat the same things over and over, usually something from the following list. I'm including this because people keep asking me about it, thinking that I don't eat much. Ha! As you'll see, I eat plenty, and it's not all what might be considered "healthy" either. I'm not suggesting that anybody eat this way, but this is what works for me...

Breakfast

- protein smoothies after strength training (protein powder, frozen fruit, green food, chia/flax seed, stevia and acai berry powder) – a custom food entered recipe into MFP
- breakfast 1-2 times a week (non strength training days) – a fried egg on half English muffin (or slice of honey wheat bread), 1 slice of bacon; I used to have cheese with this but

have gradually reduced dairy intake, so now only occasionally

- Chobani greek yogurt (occasionally)
- grapes (in the morning, my first breakfast)

Lunch

- watermelon for lunch (when in season)
- Fuji apples
- navel oranges
- chobani Greek Yogurt (when I'm not swearing off dairy)

Dinner

- 50/50 salad mix (greens plus spinach) with broiled/baked fish or chicken
- 2 boiled eggs with a can of tuna, light mayo with olive oil and mustard with a slice of honey wheat bread
- air fried catfish, shrimp, chicken wings, wingettes with steamed broccoli
- clam chowder (freshly made, never canned)
- Chopped salad w/ french bread – made with California Pizza Kitchen recipe (Google it or visit www.SharonOdom.comsoar for the recipe) – OMG it's so good!
- salmon and shrimp scampi with green beans or spinach, served over angel hair pasta w/ Parmesan cheese
- chicken chili (homemade, with beans)

- seafood gumbo (made from scratch, grandmother's recipe)

- smoked or sauteed tilapia with steamed spinach

- salmon – smoked, sauteed, baked, blackened

- baked chicken (sometimes with hot wing mix and light ranch dressing)

- french or ciabatta bread with extra virgin olive oil or olive oil infused butter (occasional treat)

- chicken enchiladas (homemade) w/ cheese, pico de gallo and a bit of light sour cream (maybe a few tablespoons of rice and beans) – this is an occasional indulgence when my weight is at the low end of the spectrum and I'm cooking dinner for the kids

Veggies

- green beans (fresh, cooked with a bit of olive oil, smoked turkey neck and creole seasoning)

- broccoli (sometimes with melted cheddar cheese)

- steamed spinach

- 50/50 salad mix (fresh greens and spinach) – add any protein and this becomes a meal

Eating Out

- occasionally a Jersey Mike's Club Sub or Schlotzsky's Smoked Turkey sandwich (pre-planned for sure – after grapes for breakfast and a hard workout)

- El Pollo Loco flame grilled chicken with flour tortillas, charro beans and broccoli – YUM! Again, this would be my main meal of the day, planned ahead of time

- Fried drum fish or catfish from my favorite hole in the wall fish place, WITH french fries (definitely my main meal of the day)

- blackened or grilled salmon or chicken salad with dressing on the side

- New York style cheese pizza by the slice – whenever I feel like it, non-negotiable (but actually not that often because of the "price" in carbs and calories; the important thing is, I can have it any time I want it, as long as I'm willing to pay the price.)

Snacks

- Yasso Greek Yogurt bars

- Whitman's Pecan Crowns

- ONE Oatmeal raisin cookie occasionally – must be fresh baked, *not* pre-packaged on aisle 7!

- Teacakes (homemade aka "Shankleville crack")

- Kind Bar (occasionally when I'm out and need to eat something)

- Sweet & salty granola bar (high in carbs, so not too often)

- Sugar free jello with a few grapes and a bit of whipped cream

- Crab ceviche (lump crab, pico de gallo, lemon juice and Uncle Chris steak seasoning), with 1 serving tortilla chips (sometimes this is lunch or dinner)

- Gorgonzola cheese with wine, grapes and crackers – YUM! (sometimes this is dinner)
- Frozen yogurt (whenever I feel like it)
- Cheese sticks (unless I'm cutting back on dairy)

Other

- Luden's sugar free cherry cough drops (for some reason I've developed a habit of sucking on these at night or on outdoor walks, trying to quit)
- A glass of white wine, usually sparkling spumante, moscato or Riesling (whenever I feel like it)
- Water in the form of decaf green tea or flavored with fruit drink mix (like crystal light)
- Daily vitamin supplements

You'll notice that except for eating out, snacks and "other", almost everything is **fresh** or **homemade**. I like to cook my own food, that way I know exactly what's in it.

My mother's family is from Louisiana, and I learned as a child how to season food well, so my cooking almost always tastes better than anything commercially prepared. It's also cheaper to cook your own meals. I don't use many canned goods, just stuff like tuna and tomato sauce.

It really boils down to focusing on more fruits, vegetables, nuts, seafood, high quality oils, lean meats, legumes (beans), quality dairy and whole grains.

Speaking of whole grains ... confessions are in order: I still eat regular angel hair pasta and french bread. Yes, I know I should eat whole wheat pasta and whole grain bread, but I don't like the taste.

I'll keep trying, but here's the thing... I'm disciplined enough in most areas, and don't eat pasta or bread that often. When I *do* have bread, I want warm slices of ciabatta or french bread with slightly toasted edges, served with balsamic vinegar and olive oil. Or olive butter. So, that's what I have – white bread, even if it means sacrificing a bit of healthiness.

Take Your Vitamins

When you restrict your food intake, it's hard to get all of the nutrients your body needs solely from eating. This is where vitamins come in. Everyone's needs are different, so you should get your doctor to come up with a vitamin plan.

I take a bunch of vitamins and supplements, including:

- Daily multivitamin
- Apple Cider Vinegar (in pill form daily)
- Eye vitamins (Lutein & Zeaxanthin)
- Pollen aid (helps with allergies)
- COQ10 – heart health
- Biotin – hair, skin and nails

A lot of medical professionals say that vitamins are a waste of money. Maybe, but I take them anyway, just in case. Again, check with your doctor about which vitamins are best for you.

Eating Out is NOT About the Food

Whenever I eat out, it's usually grilled/blackened chicken or salmon salad with the dressing on the side. Or grilled tilapia/shrimp with veggies. Even if it comes with rice or potatoes, you don't have to eat all of it. Enjoy a few bites, savor the taste, then stop. If you have trouble eating a little of something, then don't allow it on your plate. Likewise, send away the bread and chips if you can't resist. Know thyself...

All restaurants offer something healthy or grilled these days, even KFC and McDonald's. And it's easy to look up anything in MFP that you might be thinking about eating to see what it will "cost" you in calories, protein, carbs, etc.

Sure, every now and then I might have a couple fried shrimp or something I wouldn't normally eat (usually off of someone else's plate), but not much of it because it usually upsets my stomach. But it's important to know that you CAN have whatever you want.

Once your body gets used to healthy eating, it rejects the other stuff. It's really not worth it. Why eat something you don't really enjoy, then pay it for later in exercise, stomach pain, or when you see the number on the scale?

It's taken me *years* to learn that the goal of eating out is to enjoy the company of my family and friends, **NOT** to consume the most calories by eating something "good".

NO, it's **not** good, it's fattening! And if I eat it, I can't have my yogurt bar or glass of wine later on. Or I have to give up something the next day, or walk longer to make up for it. Or the next time I weigh myself, the number will be a higher than the last time. It's *always* a trade off. This is how skinny people stay that way, they just don't talk about it...

Take Food Photos

When eating out or having something you don't normally eat, **take a picture of your plate before you start eating**. That makes it easier to go back and enter the meal into MFP or whatever you're using for food logging.

Actually it's good to do it anyway, for accountability. You can post the pics to your blog, Instagram or wherever, to show what you're eating.

Oh, and here's another tip – use small plates! It's a mind trick – a little food will look like a lot.

Love Everything You Eat

I love everything that I eat, or at least like it. If not, I won't eat it. If I buy it and don't like it, into the trash it goes. Why pay twice? Just because you bought it doesn't mean you have to eat it, no matter what your mother said about not wasting food when you were growing up!

Whether it's something you or someone else brought home from the store, home cooked, or dinner out – if you're not feeling it, don't eat it. **Eat only foods you love.** If someone's feelings are hurt, oh well.

And if it means eating a delicious french baguette instead of a whole wheat roll, so be it. Don't be a slave to "healthy" eating. As long as you eat well most of the time, it all evens out.

Drink Lots of Water

If you want to lose weight, drinking water is a proven tool that's cheap, natural, calorie free and good for you. It helps to remove the hormones and toxins released when your body breaks down fat cells.

The most common recommendation is to drink at least 64 ounces per day. But like everything else, it's up to you to decide – whatever works for you. Let thirst be your guide.

If you don't like water, disguise it as tea. I make decaf green tea, sweeten with stevia, and chill it. That's my favorite version of water.

Here's another version: bottled water flavored with Airborne tablet and one of those fitness drink mixes. I still drink plain water, but prefer a little flavor.

Of course the best version is pure water, good ole H2O. Don't be like me. Drink your water straight.

This is a Game

Once you get it, that this is a game of deposits and withdrawals between your mouth and your body, it becomes easier to resist that piece of cake of whatever. If you really want it, have it, track it, and know what you're giving up in exchange.

And know that if you consistently consume the cake, the mixed drinks, the bread or whatever, without maintaining a caloric deficit, you're not going to lose weight, you'll gain. Not right away, but over time. That's how all weight losses and gains happen ... over time.

If you go off the rails, get back on track tomorrow. *Nip it in the bud right then.* Don't let it get any worse.

It all boils down to this – what are you willing to give up in return for being your desired weight? Unless you're naturally thin and have a high metabolism, this is the conversation you'll be having in your head as long as you're alive and want to stay at this weight. It's either that or be overweight.

Losing weight is hard.

Being fat is hard.

Choose your hard.

Step #5: Embrace Exercise

Alright, here we go. Let's get this out of the way. If you want to lose weight and feel great doing it, you're going to have to embrace exercise. Sorry if that's not what you want to hear, but it's the truth. You must embrace exercise or it's going to be a long hard road to fitness.

Sorry, but there's no way to sugarcoat it. If you want to lose weight without exercising, be prepared to eat very little and feel deprived.

Although <u>it's possible to lose weight without exercising, it will</u>

take a lot longer to reach your goal. Sure you can lose weight but you're going to be hungry, flabby and irritable.

Plus, exercise will help you look and feel better along the way. Also, time spent exercising is time you're not eating! And there's something about exercising that makes you want to eat healthy.

No Excuses

Here's a common excuse: I don't have time to exercise. Maybe, but if you get sick, you'll make the time to go to the doctor, right? You may think that you're healthy, but truth is, if you're overweight, you just haven't gotten sick yet. Eventually it will probably catch up with you.

All I know is this: every time I come down with a cold, headache or backache, *anything* that leaves me feeling less than 100%, it's a reminder that ...

Health is your greatest wealth. As long as you have your health, ***anything*** **is possible.**

If you have your health, *you are wealthy beyond measure.* There are rich people who would trade places with you in an instant. They would give you every cent of their money to get what you have – good health.

And if you want to keep that good health, get off your ass and use what God has given you, while you still can!

The good news is that it doesn't take that much exercise to have a positive impact, especially if you haven't been doing any. You just have to decide that you're going to commit to exercise as part of your life plan. Then make the time to do it. Even a 20 minute daily walk can make a difference.

By the way, if it truly is a challenge for you to find the time to exercise, there are all sorts of ways to burn calories even when you're not exercising per se. Again, look up Dr. James Levine and the concept of NEAT, you'll see what I mean. Things like taking the stairs, not looking for the closest parking place, knee bends while talking on the phone. In other words, keep your body in motion. Your body will thank you.

So the question is, what is this going to look like for you? Like the food plan, your exercise plan has to be **specific to you,** customized for you, fit into your life seamlessly. Something you enjoy doing, or at least that you don't mind doing.

What's Your Favorite Workout

Do you like to walk? Jog? Bike ride? Play tennis? Swim? Skate? Lift weights? Have sex? Hey, that can be good exercise! What do you *truly* enjoy doing that will burn off some calories?

C'mon, there's got to be something that you like to do to move your body. Anything. It doesn't matter. But it needs to be something that you can do easily and often. Mix it up. Walk some days, other days go biking. Just do *something*.

You know by now that I've burned countless calories since 2006 without even thinking about it on my treadmill desk. It was definitely the biggest tool in my weight loss toolbox. If you like walking and have the space for it, I encourage you to get your own treadmill desk.

But if a treadmill desk is not for you, what about an exercise bike desk? Yes a desk with a stationary bike attached! There are tons of options when it comes to home gym equipment. As technology has improved, it's even easier now to create the exact workout setup you need, including for very small spaces. It's amazing how so many things are collapsible, foldable and "slidable" these days.

The reason I put such an emphasis on having your own equipment is simple – I don't like schlepping to the gym, waiting for equipment, or anything else about it. But if you like working out at a gym and will go regularly, great. The point is to find what works for you. Some people hate working out at home and can only exercise in a gym setting. Whatever works, as long as it's something you'll do on a regular basis.

Mindless Exercise

Try to find a form of exercise that you like or at least don't mind doing. For me, that thing was walking. It's the easiest thing to do, all you need is a good pair of walking shoes and a place to walk. Or a treadmill, which is what I use most of the time. Thanks to my treadmill desk, walking was already a habit. And even better, it was **mindless exercise**.

What's mindless exercise? It's exercise that you can do without thinking, while you're doing something else. Like walking or jogging on your treadmill desk, or peddling on your stationary bike. These are activities you can do at home anytime, rain or shine.

It's perfect for taking your mind off the fact that you're exercising while you watch TV, surf the internet, talk on the phone, whatever.

Oh, and if you work at home and are in control of your environment then you have NO excuse! Likewise, if you're retired and don't have to be anywhere every day, no excuse. If you work at a job every day, yes it could be challenging to walk every day. But you can do it.

Once I started eating right, the exercise took everything to the next level. I joined the Fitbit community to find out why my device didn't accurately measure steps on the treadmill. From there I met others, made Fitbit friends, and began to join challenges. The competitions are just for fun, but there's something about seeing how you compare to others that makes you walk a little farther. The camaraderie and encouragement is really a motivator, at least it was for me.

Maybe that doesn't appeal to you – again, **it's about finding what works for you.** There has to be something that you like doing that will burn calories. It doesn't even have to make you sweat. What is it?

Another form of mindless exercise is not really exercise at all. I touched upon it earlier. It's called NEAT (Non-Exercise Activity Thermogenesis), which was pioneered by Dr. James Levine, a Mayo clinic obesity researcher.

NEAT is the energy expended or calories burned for everything we do that is not sleeping, eating, or sports-like exercise. These activities can be anything that involves movement – housework, gardening, puttering, fidgeting, standing, basically anything other than sitting. Being active increases your metabolic rate, so keep your body moving!

Track Your Exercise

In December 2015 my daughter Mariah and I went to Verizon to get new phones. Christmas was coming up and when Mimi traded in her phone, she got a Fitbit for me as part of her trade-in package. Little did I know how much it would come to mean to me.

At the time I hadn't started my weight loss journey. I was almost 220 pounds and knew that eventually I'd have to do something to stem the tide of weight gain. So when she gave me the Fitbit for Christmas I was like, cool. I can use this to track my steps. I put it on my wrist and didn't think too much about it.

Then came February 1st, 2016, the day I got serious. We had commemorated the one year anniversary of my Mom's passing on January 15th. I decided to get my ass in gear and knew food logging and exercise tracking would be crucial.

I linked MyFitnessPal and Fitbit so they could exchange data. From then on all steps logged by Fitbit were passed to MFP and tracked as exercise. By logging everything I eat in MFP and keeping an eye on the Fitbit calories, I started maintaining a **daily deficit of 1,000 calories**.

If it was late in the day and the deficit wasn't 1,000, I simply went for a walk or got on the treadmill desk to watch TV, surf the internet, work, or talk on the phone.

Given a choice between not eating something delicious or walking to earn it, I'll choose walking every time. It's worth it to be able to eat whatever I want! For me, this is key – **no deprivation, no hunger pangs, nothing off limits.**

There are other fitness trackers, and of course there are phone apps that can track your activity. But because my daughter gave me a Fitbit, that's the one I use. In case it's not abundantly clear, Fitbit has been a **huge** part of my success.

You can track any type of exercise in Fitbit and other trackers so my question to you is... how do you like to move your body?

MyFitnessPal + Fitbit

The combination of **MFP** for food tracking and **Fitbit** for exercise tracking was *magic* for me. Something about using these two tools together *clicked*. MFP syncs with Fitbit so you can see at a glance where you are as far as your calorie deficit.

MFP syncs with other fitness trackers, and of course there are other food logging programs out there as well. But MFP and Fitbit are the ones that I use, and I love them both! Both of the apps are free, the only cost is the Fitbit tracker itself.

At first I used to enter exercise manually into Fitbit, afraid it wouldn't give me credit for every little calorie burned. Too much work. Eventually I stopped doing that, and just let Fitbit figure out how many calories I burned and send it to MFP. If it underestimates a bit, oh well.

I don't even bother entering my strength training workouts. Too much work. That is my built in cushion, in case I underestimate the calories entered into MFP.

You might prefer other tools than MFP and Fitbit, but tracking your *input* and *output* is vital for getting a handle on what's going on with your body.

Step #6: Be Accountable

Losing weight can be a lonely journey, especially if you don't have enough support. Who knows whether you're hitting your goals or not? Who will you talk to when you're stuck on a plateau, or when you feel like you're never going to reach your goal?

Yes, motivation is an inside job, and it's largely up to you to hold onto that vision of you at your ideal weight. In my case, my conviction was so strong that being accountable solely to myself was plenty. I'd promised my mother, even though she wasn't alive to witness it. And I'd promised myself. That was enough.

But sometimes you need support. If you're going it alone, not to worry – there are plenty of resources for you. Trust me, you will NOT be alone on this journey unless you choose to be.

And when it comes to weight loss, you won't find a larger group (pardon the pun) of people who are in the same boat as you. If you want to be held accountable for your fitness goals, you have plenty of options.

Find Your Clique

If you join a weight loss program that has in-person meetings, that's a great source of support. Most programs now have online support forums for members. Those are great places to find workout buddies and connect with others facing the same challenges. Other options include...

- **MyFitnessPal** - the food logging tool is only part of what MFP offers, you also get access to an online community of like minded people of all ages, from all over the world. Members share weight loss tips, success stories and helpful comments. Best of all, it's free.

- **Fitbit** – this community consists of Fitbit forums (online) and Fitbit friends (app) who you step with during Fitbit challenges. You'll end up with a regular "clique" of people you step with and your virtual workout buddies will cheer you on.

- **Instagram.com** – My cousin Angelique (@angeliquemiles) is a major star on IG. Every time she posts something it gets thousands of likes. Me? Not so much. I'd heard of it but didn't really use it much until I reached goal. What a mistake that was on my part! Instagram is wonderful for weight loss stories and transformations. I SO wish that I had posted to IG from day 1. It's such a welcoming friendly place, everybody is so encouraging. Highly recommended. People will cheer you on, guaranteed. Take your "Before" picture and post it on Day #1. Then keep going. Start posting every day, it will create a record of your journey. You'll develop a following, your own clique. Use hashtags so people can find you. Post as if you have a large audience, even if you don't – one day you will, and all of your posts will still be there for them to like, comment on, etc. Instagram is awesome!   **(@sharoneodom)**

- **Facebook** – there are many groups dedicated to weight loss, where people meet and encourage each other in their weight loss and fitness pursuits.

- **Friends** – don't overlook your IN PERSON real life friends. Is there someone you know, a friend, girlfriend, cousin perhaps – that could stand to lose 25 or 50 pounds? Or whatever amount you need to lose. Sometimes all you need is that small push...

If all else fails, you'll have to rely on the **one** person you can *really* count on – yourself. You made a pact with yourself. Lie to others if you must but not to yourself.

You are accountable first and foremost … to you. That's what matters. Figure out your accountability system. Even if it's just to yourself.

Step #7: Stay Motivated

Remember what I said about weight loss being more mental than physical? Here's where that comes into play.

Weight loss begins in your mind. When you finally experience "the click" that inspired the title of this book, something happens inside that makes it possible for you to do what you were unable to do before. No matter how many times you've tried.

This is why knowing your "why" is so important. *Why* do you want to lose weight in the first place? How important it is to you? What you're willing to give up to get it? You have to be *absolutely clear* in your mind about all of these things.

Above all, you must have a vision of yourself at your goal weight. If you have an actual picture of yourself at your ideal weight (like my "girl on the fence" picture), by all means post it on your refrigerator.

Or create a **vision board** of what your life will look at at your goal weight and put it there.

When the going gets tough, you'll need to be able to dig down deep, draw on your inner reserves, and hold onto that picture of yourself at a healthy weight.

That **inner seeing**, *inner knowing*, that vision of your life in your new body --- those are the things that will get you through any setback or weight loss plateau.

The Dreaded Weight Loss Plateau

In the first year, my weight loss averaged about 1.5 lbs per week, but it was *not* a straight line. Some weeks it was nothing or even a slight gain.

Other times 4-5 pounds would melt away within a week. As I discussed earlier, this is called the **"whoosh-bounce-hold"** cycle: a big loss one week, followed by a small bounce back, a pound or two, followed by holding relatively steady for another week or two.

Weight fluctuations are normal. Your weight can vary 1 to 3 pounds daily depending on a lot of things, including salt and water intake. That's one reason I don't usually weigh myself every day, although some people swear by it. Whatever works for you...

Initially my regular weigh-in day was Sunday, but after my first whoosh-bounce-hold cycle, I modified it to continue the weigh-ins but **only record a loss in MFP**. If the number on the scale was bigger than the last weigh-in, I simply did not record it. To me that was too demoralizing.

I made a note of it in my journal, but refused to acknowledge it officially. But I made sure not to do this too often. Again, this was MY rule, it's what worked for me. You might consider that to be cheating. Well, if I were following somebody else's plan it might be, which is why you should *find what works for you!*

I couldn't go too long without recording my weight, so that made me work extra hard the next week so I could record a loss. Yes, a crooked line is more realistic than a straight path but I didn't want to see any upticks. That's why my weight loss journey doesn't show any, but believe me, they happened. And like I said earlier, eventually I got over that foolishness and accepted weight fluctuations as normal, **which they are**.

Set Milestones Along the Way

Having a big end goal is great, but you're not going to get there overnight. It's important for your psyche and your motivation to get encouragement along the way in the form of milestones, with rewards for hitting them.

In my case, I set a mini goal every few pounds from the time I started til I reached goal, and even beyond. Each step represented something I wanted to accomplish, and it gave me something to look forward to in the near term instead of months away.

From the beginning, here are the mini goals I had to look forward to all along the way.

- Start: 222.5 (BMI 35.9)
- get under 220 (BMI 35.3)
- get to BMI under 35 (216.0)
- 210, only 10 pounds away from the 190s
- Next weight goal - 200.0, then 199.5
- Then...185-186 -- new BMI threshold (from obese to overweight)
- Also 185 is the HALFWAY point to 148
- 180 pounds, then 179
- 172.5 - 50 lbs lost
- 170, then 169
- 162.5 - 60 lost

- 161 - 61 lbs lost

- Then, 158, my lowest weight since the triplets were born

- 154.5 - normal weight

- 152.5 - 70 lbs lost

- THEN 150, then...

- 149 – finally under 150

- 148!!! - lost 1/3 body weight

Yes, it seems a little ridiculous, but those mini milestones kept it interesting, and gave me something to look forward to every few pounds.

How did I reward myself? With small extravagances like a manicure/pedicure, facial, massage. New workout clothes. A trip to Los Angeles for my birthday to celebrate losing 80 pounds. A new car at the 90 pound mark.

The more I lost, the higher the value went up, rewarding myself with things I wouldn't normally buy. Heck, even if it's something I *would* buy, like a mani/pedi, this way forced me to "earn" it. Oh, the games you have to play with yourself...

As I got closer to goal, my favorite rewards became … cute little outfits in sizes 6-8. There's nothing like shopping for clothes in single digit sizes when you've been buying sizes 18-22 for so long!

Don't Eat Your Feelings

This is a tough one, something I still struggle with to this day. It's so easy to eat your feelings when everything is going wrong. Or you're bored.

Listen, from babyhood we learn to associate food with love, safety, and comfort. As kids we're often rewarded or bribed with food.

Think of how we celebrate special occasions throughout our lives – food. It's no wonder that we turn to food to soothe and comfort ourselves. As my daughter says, "Food does not disappoint."

Food is also a great way to distract ourselves from the crap going on in our lives. When reviewing my journal I noticed patterns – those times when I was more likely to fall off the wagon.

Stress over the impending move led to scarfing more teacakes. Frustration over my kids' life choices sent me running for the fried fish. Thoughts about my love life called for a trip to the pizza place. And an extra glass of wine.

There's something intoxicating about comfort food. It's easy to unconsciously suck down thousands of calories and not even remember it.

Well, it might feel good in the moment, but like the worst hangover, you'll feel like crap afterwards. Especially when you visit the scale. And whatever emotional stuff you were trying to bury under all that food and drink will still be there.

So what can we do to comfort ourselves besides eat? Lots of things!

First, think about when you're most likely to overindulge. If you keep a journal, review it for patterns. You might gain some insight into what is likely to send you diving into the nearest cake. Figure out your emotional triggers.

If you feel a binge coming on, pick up the phone and call a friend for some emotional nourishment. Pace or walk around while you're on the phone. The treadmill desk is great for getting exercise while talking on the phone or watching TV...

If all your friends are busy, go for a walk. Exercise is a natural anti-depressant and it burns calories. Win-win!

Don't feel like walking? Listen to some music. Read a book. Vacuum the house. Do laundry. Treat yourself to a massage. Do something – anything – to distract yourself from the hum of the refrigerator.

If you decide to indulge, do it mindfully. Controlled portions of favorite comfort foods works – buy ONE oatmeal raisin cookie from Whole Foods and savor every crumb. Or **one** package of pecan turtles, one of my favorites.

Eating your feelings is part of being human. Just know that you can comfort yourself in ways that won't derail your success or make you feel bad. Come up with your own coping mechanisms **ahead of time** so that you'll be ready.

And if you do succumb, dust yourself off and get back on it!

Stress Can Derail Weight Loss

Closely related to eating your feelings is *stress*, which is usually why you eat your feelings in the first place. So let's talk about that – how does stress affect weight loss?

As it turns out, stress is the #1 reason that people gain weight so it stands to reason it could play a big part in the battle to lose weight.

Here's the thing - when you're stressed out, nothing else really matters, at least not to your body. When you're buried underneath stress, everything seems harder. If you try to lose weight while constantly stressed out, your body's nervous system becomes overloaded.

That's because stress produces the hormone **cortisol**, which has been known to trigger cravings for comfort foods. Stress also increases **insulin** levels, which impedes your ability to burn off those comfort foods.

The combination of increased cortisol and insulin levels is a double whammy – it sends strong signals to fat cells to hold onto their fat stores, because your body thinks you need those extra calories to deal with the stress.

This amounts to fighting your body, which can make it *really* hard to lose weight. Sure you can do it, but stress makes everything a lot harder than it needs to be.

We all have a limited amount of time and energy. When we have to use these resources to deal with stressful situations or their aftermath, that leaves a lot less time for healthy habits.

Stress that goes on for a long period increases your appetite, makes your body hold onto fat and takes away the willpower you need to maintain a healthy lifestyle.

In other words, when you're stressed, it's easier to give in to food cravings and skip workouts. It's harder to get enough sleep and plan healthy meals. All of this only adds to your stress. It's a vicious cycle that you must break.

Managing Stress

Life happens. We all have to deal with stress, but if we manage it well, there's no reason those little bumps in the road have to derail our weight loss program.

So what's the answer? First, admit that you're stressed. It took me a long time to recognize the effect that stress had on my weight, and even longer to get it under control. Once I made a conscious effort to remove the stressors in my life, I was able to focus on losing weight.

When you make your health a priority and find ways to cope that don't involve stuffing your face, you can free up the emotional energy needed to reduce stress.

Once you do that, you'll be able to devote more energy to exercise, plan healthy meals, and get enough sleep. Losing weight will become a whole lot easier. This is what happens when you start to work with your body instead of fighting yourself every step of the way.

Make time for leisure and hobbies, which have been shown to reduce stress. Hiking became one of my favorite hobbies, which certainly helped my weight loss efforts. But I also like travel, creative writing, and photography. Self care can take many forms, so if you like painting, pottery or gardening, go for it.

Finally, try to begin and end your day with calm and relaxation, perhaps a few minutes of meditation, yoga, or journaling. Winding down at the end of the day can help you sleep better, and just maybe will help tomorrow feel a little less stressful.

Step #8: Maintain, Don't Gain

Maintenance is a 4 letter word. Pick your 4 letter word.

This is where most weight loss stories hit the skids. Why? Because it's so damn hard! Ask me how I know this...

You can do anything for a short period of time, which is about how long most "diets" last. As soon as they're over, the weight returns.

This is the cycle you have to break ... now. This is what "**The Click**" is all about.

It's when you realize that *this is it*. **This is your new lifestyle,** and you embrace it. You decide to forever change the way you eat and exercise. And you must, or else the old you will return. For sure.

I remember all too well how it feels to be big and wear size 2XL. And the bigger I got, the more invisible I felt. It wasn't all that long ago, so the memory is still fresh. Not to mention all those embarrassing "before" pics.

That's a feeling I NEVER want to have again.

Embrace Maintenance

So, I embrace maintenance the same way we embrace brushing our teeth, taking showers, or going to the doctor or dentist for checkups. Not something you love, but you do because it's part of staying healthy.

If I want to continue to wear cute little size 6-8 outfits, maintenance is a must. The reality is, to keep the weight off, you need to make permanent changes to your lifestyle.

Here's the good thing. I've found a way of life that lets me eat all the foods I love. I'm genuinely happy with my body, so maintenance is a small price to pay. Once you get used to leaping out of bed in the morning instead of lumbering, you never want to go back. Yes, it's a pain in the ass to count calories and exercise. But so is being overweight. Both are hard. Choose your hard.

Actually the hardest part of maintenance is figuring out the balance between losing and gaining weight. It's something I'm not accustomed to because frankly, all of my adult like I've been either losing weight *or* gaining weight. One or the other.

Now I'm not trying to lose weight unless I've gained a few pounds. What a feeling! It's definitely foreign to me and most yo-yo dieters. You have to learn a whole new way of being – steady state. Neither losing nor gaining. And if you go off rails, just get back on track tomorrow. Don't let things get out of hand. Better to nip it in the bud when you have 2 or 5 pounds to lose – don't wait til you have 20. Or 50. Or 90. Been there. Done that. No way I'm going back.

PART IV:

FINAL THOUGHTS

Some final thoughts that didn't fit anywhere else...

Things People Say

When you lose a significant amount of weight, every conversation you have with people who knew the overweight you will be about your new body. This will go on for awhile.

"Wow, you look great!"

"How much have you lost?"

"How did you do it?"

"You're going to get anorexia!"

You'll get lots of questions and compliments. Some of them will be backhand compliments. Some will imply that you'll probably gain it all back. Ignore them all.

The best response to everybody is to say thank you and change the subject. If someone presses the issue or really wants to know how you did it so they can do it too, tell them. Most people will lose interest pretty quickly.

Here's the thing – very few people want to hear the truth. That there is no secret to weight loss. That you must count calories and move your ass. That's not sexy. That's not the magic bullet that everybody's looking for. There's nothing you can do about that so don't even try.

The funniest thing is when they watch what you put on your plate. They're always shocked when I have a piece of cake. Of course they don't want to hear that I walked 20,000 steps beforehand and banked my calories so I could splurge.

Beware of Saboteurs

For the most part you'll find people are supportive of your weight loss journey, but beware … you will run across some haters.

These could be friends, family, co-workers or perfect strangers. They are people who have decided that it's their business what you put in your mouth.

Some of these people are jealous because you're making changes they wish they could make. Maybe it's a thin friend who loves having a fat friend around to make her look better. Or an overweight friend who likes having another fattie for company.

Whatever. Fact is, you're the only person who's affected by what you eat. It's your body and your life. Practice saying "I'm not hungry", or "I just ate". If you worry about hurting people's feelings, learn to push food around on your plate and pretend you're eating it. Or throw it away when nobody's looking.

Personally I've learned to happily ignore all external input. I eat or not eat exactly what I please, with no apologies or explanations necessary. And so should you. Anybody else's opinion means nothing. Even if it comes from your husband and/or children.

Clothes Shopping Is Fun

When you're overweight, shopping for clothes can be a miserable experience. Nothing looks good. Things cost more. Most of them are ugly. The selection is so limited that if you find anything that halfway fits and looks remotely decent, you buy it.

After weight loss, a whole new world opens up to you. No more prowling the plus size section in the back corner of the store. You have the entire store to choose from. *Everything* is in your size. In multiple colors.

You no longer have to buy something just because it fits. You have *lots* of choices, and can even find cute stuff on sale. *In your size.* Gorgeous clothes are everywhere, for cheap. Check out thrift stores.

Forget about the baggy look. That was for the fat you. Think fitted. The thin you wants to show off a little. Refuse to wear anything that doesn't make you look and feel fabulous.

You worked hard for your new body, there's nothing wrong with being a little bit vain. Go on, celebrate. Dress as if you're proud of yourself. It's one of the best rewards for losing all that weight.

Losing Weight Does Not Solve All of Your Problems

I *love* my life now. Is it perfect? No. All of your problems won't magically disappear just because you lose weight. Life doesn't suddenly become a bed of roses. That's a fallacy that many overweight people believe. That all their problems will melt away with the fat. It doesn't work that way.

Being overweight is a great excuse for being unhappy. But what happens when the fat is gone? Now what's your excuse for not accomplishing everything you want to do with your life? That's when you have to confront the underlying problems, all of the crap in your life that you blamed on being overweight.

Whatever problems you have at 225 pounds will likely still await you at 135 pounds. But being overweight won't be one of them. There are a whole lot of good reasons to be happy about this, but at the end of it all, you're still left with … you.

This sucks. You go through hell and back to lose the weight, only to find out that fat was only part of the problem. Now you have to deal with the rest of it. Don't be surprised when this happens.

But it's still worth it to lose the weight, if for no other reason than you'll feel better, look better, and stand a better chance of being around to experience all the other joys that life has in store for you. You'll also have a heightened sense of self-belief. Remember, you lost all that weight. If you can do that, you can do anything.

My Life Today

I've been at a normal weight since December 2016, when I reached 154.5. Once I achieved my goal of 148 pounds, I started weight training, and lost another 15 pounds.

Today my weight fluctuates between 131 and 136. I monitor it weekly, and make whatever adjustments necessary to stay around 135. That's my target. Maybe one day I'll go for 129, just for fun ... and re-create that "girl on the fence" picture!

Sometimes I eat more, exercise less, and gain a few pounds as a result. Yes, I do fall off the wagon at times, especially during the summer.

But I've learned to react the same way a normal person would –

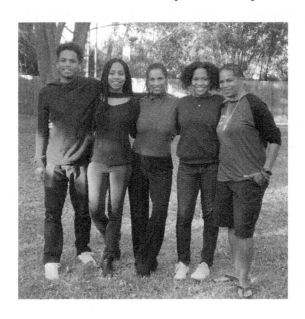

"Oops, I've gained a few pounds, better cut back." Not, "OMG! I've gained 10 pounds, I'm a failure!" That all or nothing thinking is the road back to obesity.

Life happens, and food is an easy crutch for emotional eaters. Acknowledge it, let go of the guilt, and figure out what's behind the weight gain. Then take corrective measures.

When it happens, I've learned to put on the brakes, pull back to about 1,300 calories a day, increase my exercise, and create the caloric deficit needed to lose those few pounds.

It usually only takes a few days to see results, and it feels so good to know that things are not out of control. Having 3 or 4 pounds to lose is *way* better than 20, 40... or 90.

I've learned to accept that I will *always* struggle with food – wanting more of it than my body needs. Knowing that if I give into those desires consistently, I'll be fat again.

I don't profess to have all the answers, but this I know – I've come too far to fall off the wagon and stay off. No matter what, I have no choice but to climb back on.

Am I out of the woods yet? No, not by a long shot. But I've learned a lot, and like my chances. For one thing, all of my fat clothes are gone. Donated or thrown away.

Not only that, I've written this book, telling the whole world about how I lost 90 pounds. After sharing those mortifying "before" pictures, I'm *very* motivated to do whatever it takes to keep it off.

I've faced the fact that maintenance will **always** be a part of my life, which is why it's so important to create a plan that you can follow… for life. But I *love* being this size, and that's way more important to me than sitting on my ass stuffing my face.

It's Your Turn …

Ok, it's your turn. Everything you need to lose weight is within your grasp. You can do it, *if* you're ready. Really *mentally* ready.

How do you know when you're ready? Many weight loss stories start the same way mine did, with something resembling "the click".

There are many terms for it – the moment, the straw, rock bottom, paradigm shift, wake-up call, fed up, awakening, epiphany, pain point, dog on the tack – but they all refer to a *defining moment* that makes you realize that you are DONE. **Finished**. No more status quo.

Something happens. Something in your psyche shifts and changes. And you finally decide to do something about whatever it is. This is *not* just about weight loss. The click can be a metaphor for anything that you need to change in your life.

When you reach the point where you are no longer willing to tolerate the way you are living, you have no other choice but to change your life. Something has to change, and *it begins in your mind*. When you're ready, you'll experience "the click". That's when you start.

If weight loss is your goal, the steps have been laid out for you. All the information you need is at your fingertips. All you have to do is… start. Pick a day, hop aboard, and get going.

But remember, you're not on your own. There are tons of people ready to support you on this journey because they are going through it too. Seek and yee shall find. MyFitnessPal, Fitbit, Instagram,

Facebook, it's all right there at your fingertips – all the support you could ever need, for weight loss or whatever you want to achieve.

Just One More Thing …

Thank you for reading. If you enjoyed this book, please, **please** leave a review on Amazon! It will go a long way toward helping others discover this book and benefit from it, not to mention it will make me so very happy. Here's the review link:

http://www.amazon.com/review/create-review? &asin=**0971897115** or go here:

https://sharonodom.com/LeaveAmazonReview/

Contact Me:

You can reach me here:

- **Email**: InTheClickZone@gmail.com
- **Instagram**: @sharoneodom
- **Facebook**: Remember you are not alone on your weight loss journey. Please join us in **The Click Zone Facebook Group,** which I created to provide a safe place to discuss your weight loss struggles and get support.

  https://www.facebook.com/groups/TheClickZone
- **Website**: Visit www.SharonOdom.com for news, updates, and your FREE e-guide "Living the Click".

Made in the USA
Middletown, DE
18 September 2021

48500126R10109